Ultrasound-Guided Limb Surgery

Olivier Marès
Francisco Javier Ferreira
Julien Beldame
Editors

Ultrasound-Guided Limb Surgery

Springer

Editors
Olivier Marès
Department of Traumatology and Orthopedic Surgery
University Hospital Nîmes
Nîmes, France

Francisco Javier Ferreira
Hospital Universitario San Rafael
Madrid, Spain

Julien Beldame
Institut de la cheville et du pied
Amiens, Polyclinique de Picardie
Amiens, France

ISBN 978-3-031-88678-2 ISBN 978-3-031-88679-9 (eBook)
https://doi.org/10.1007/978-3-031-88679-9

Original French edition: "L'échochirurgie du membre supérieur" published by Sauramps Médical 2021.

This Springer imprint is published by the registered company Springer Nature Switzerland AG
The registered company address is: Gewerbestrasse 11, 6330 Cham, Switzerland

Preface

Orthopedic surgery has witnessed significant advancements with the introduction of ultrasound-guided surgery, a technique that has revolutionized the way surgeons approach diagnosis, surgical planning, and intervention execution. In this context, it becomes imperative to have a comprehensive and up-to-date book that focuses specifically on ultrasound-guided surgery in the realm of orthopedic surgery. This book, titled "Ultrasound-Guided Limb Surgery" aims to provide healthcare professionals, students, and residents with a comprehensive guide.

The importance of this book lies in its ability to address a significant gap in the current medical literature by exclusively focusing on ultrasound-guided surgery in the field of orthopedics and traumatology. As these techniques become more widely adopted, it is crucial to have a reliable and up-to-date reference that covers key aspects of this specialty. The authors, experts in the fields of orthopedic surgery and ultrasound, have compiled and synthesized the most relevant and current information, providing readers with a deep and practical understanding of this technique.

This book is as an essential tool for healthcare professionals seeking to incorporate ultrasound-guided surgery into their clinical practice. Through a combination of descriptive text, illustrations, and photographs, it delves into the various applications of ultrasound in orthopedic surgery, such as anatomical structure localization, implant placement guidance, and intraoperative evaluation. Furthermore, it addresses the challenges and limitations of the technique, as well as ethical and safety considerations.

In summary, "Ultrasound-Guided Limb Surgery" is a fundamental work that aims to stimulate interest and curiosity in the field of ultrasound-guided surgery. Its comprehensive content, practical approach, and scientific rigor make it an indispensable reference for healthcare professionals and researchers in this field.

We hope that this book will prove to be a valuable resource in both training and clinical practice, contributing to the advancement and improvement of healthcare in the field of orthopedic surgery through the use of ultrasound.

Welcome to this fascinating journey into the world of ultrasound-guided surgery in orthopedics!

Nîmes, France Olivier Marès
Madrid, Spain Francisco Javier Ferreira
Amiens, France Julien Beldame

Contents

Part I

Introduction/Basics

1 Basic Ultrasound for Ultrasound Guidance

Fernando Corella, Montserrat Ocampos, Manuel Pérez España, and Carlos Collado

1.1 Basics for Ultrasound Surgery

In the context of hand interventionism, the strategic integration of ultrasound (US) technology is of great relevance for diagnostic and therapeutic purposes. This chapter scrutinizes the nuanced dimensions of ultrasound preparation and the diverse spectrum of transducer technologies employed within the field. A comprehensive understanding of ultrasound parameters, including frequency, depth, focus adjustment, gain, and Doppler mode, is imperative for practitioners seeking to optimize their interventions.

1.1.1 Ultrasound Setup/Image Optimization for Surgery

The wise selection of the US machine, appropriate transducer, and meticulous configuration of ultrasound settings are pivotal steps in achieving optimal imaging outcomes.

1.1.2 Ultrasound Machine

The choice of a US machine is critical, taking into account features such as imaging modes, user interface, and compatibility with specific transducers. Currently, there are fixed, portable, and ultra-portable US machines, with the latter enabling wireless connections with tablets or mobile phones (Fig. 1.1).

Ultraportable devices offer advantages in terms of cost and portability, but they may not provide the same image quality as bigger and more advance ultrasound machines and face the disadvantage of potential connection loss and battery depletion during procedures.

F. Corella (✉)
Orthopedic and Trauma Department, Hospital Universitario Infanta Leonor, Madrid, Spain

Orthopedic and Trauma Department, Hospital Universitario Quironsalud Madrid, Madrid, Spain

Surgery Department, School of Medicine, Universidad Complutense de Madrid, Madrid, Spain
e-mail: fernando.corella@gmail.es

M. Ocampos · C. Collado
Orthopedic and Trauma Department, Hospital Universitario Infanta Leonor, Madrid, Spain

Orthopedic and Trauma Department, Hospital Universitario Quironsalud Madrid, Madrid, Spain

M. P. España
Orthopedic and Trauma Department, Hospital Universitario Infanta Leonor, Madrid, Spain

Orthopedic and Trauma Department, Hospital Viamed Santa Elena, Madrid, Spain

O. Marès et al. (eds.), *Ultrasound-Guided Limb Surgery*,
https://doi.org/10.1007/978-3-031-88679-9_1

1.1.3 Transducer

Before carrying out an ultrasound-guided procedure, it is important to select the most appropriate probe.

Linear transducers prove to be the most useful for the hand, wrist, and forearm, as they enable a more accurate evaluation of structures close to the skin. They operate within frequencies between 5 and 20 MHz, in contrast to curvilinear transducers that utilize frequencies between 3.5 and 5 MHz (more suitable for studying deep structures such as the hip). Matricial linear probes play a vital role in improving the imaging capacity of traditional probes in MSK ultrasound. Although clinical MSK ultrasound has traditionally utilized high-frequency probes up to 18 to 20 MHz, which are limited to superficial depths below the skin, incorporating matricial linear probes can greatly enhance both imaging depth and resolution. This enables more thorough evaluations of musculoskeletal structure.

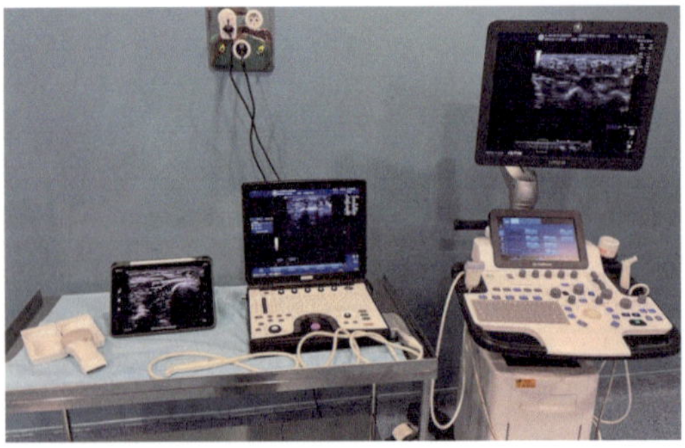

Fig. 1.1 Different types of ultrasound machines used in ultrasound-guided surgery

For procedures in the finger and hand, the hockey stick probe is the most effective, given its 2 cm footprint. The compact design of the probe allows for precise manipulation and exploration of tissues in small spaces, ensuring contact with the phalanges even with a flexed finger. Conversely, for procedures in the wrist or forearm where greater depth and a wider field of vision are necessary, a conventional linear probe is commonly used (Fig. 1.2).

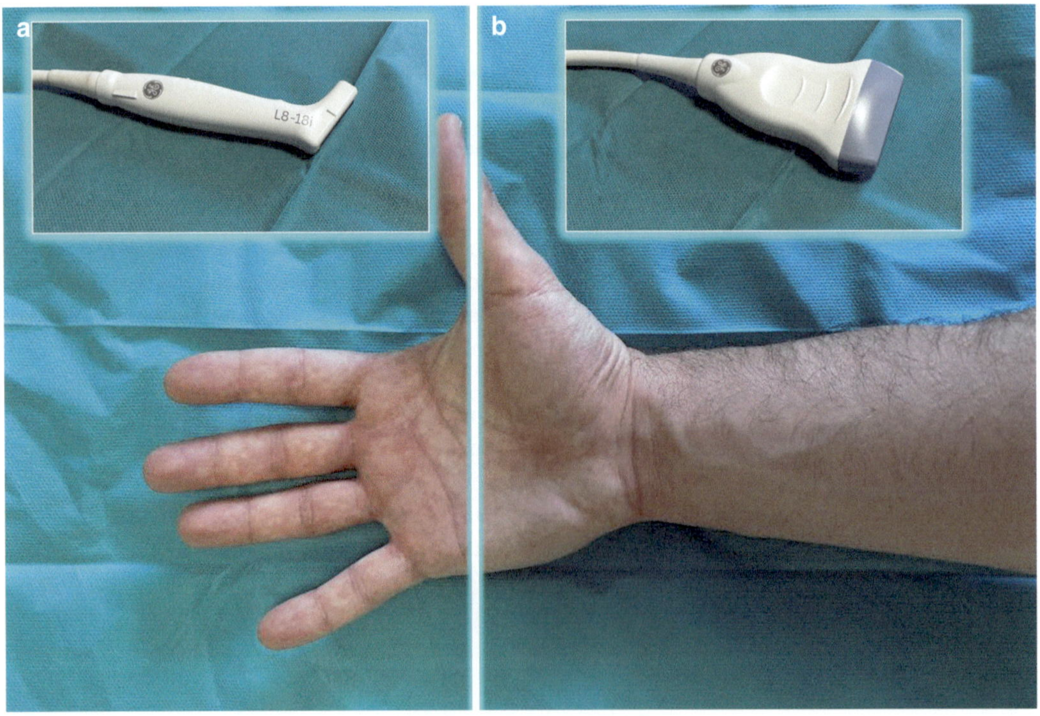

Fig. 1.2 (**a**) "Hockey stick probe". (**b**) Conventional linear probe

1.1.4 Frequency

The judicious selection of ultrasound frequency is critical, as it influences both image resolution and penetration depth.

High frequency: Conductive to superior resolution of superficial hand structures. Optimal for visualizing minute details, such as nerves and small vessels.

Low frequency: Penetrates deep tissues proficiently. Well-suited for imaging larger hand structures like joints and deep vessels.

Given that most structures in hand and wrist surgery are close to the skin, high frequencies are most useful. This high frequency enables higher resolution of nearby structures, albeit at the expense of reduced depth and penetration capabilities.

1.1.5 Depth and Focus Adjustment

1.1.5.1 Depth Adjustment

Governing the extent of the imaging field, influences the visualization of specific structures. The average depth for visualizing finger and hand structures is 1.5 to 3 cm, while the average depth in the wrist and forearm is 1.5 to 5 cm (Fig. 1.3c).

1.1.5.2 Focus Adjustment

Enables practitioners to concentrate the US beam at a defined depth, augmenting image clarity and resolution at the designated focal point. Given the narrow depth spectrum in the fingers, hand, and forearm, a single focus is typically sufficient, while in deeper structures such as the thigh or hip, two or three focuses are recommendable. It is advisable to position the focus at the place of interest or slightly below it (Fig. 1.3a–b).

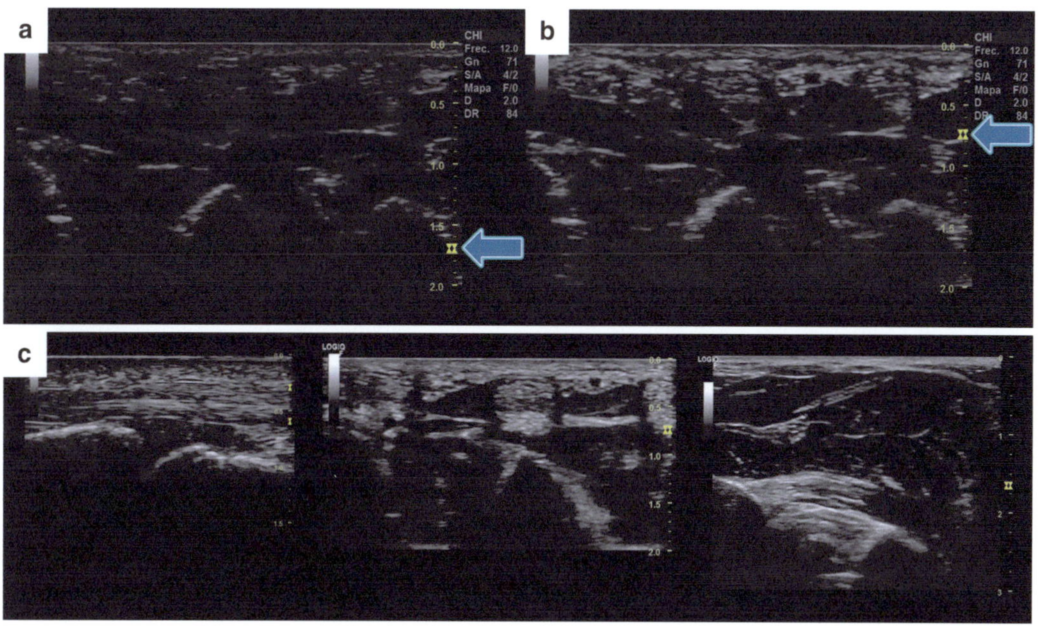

Fig. 1.3 (**a**, **b**) Location of the focus while performing an ultrasound scanning. (**c**) Examples of focus adjustment

1.1.6 Gain

The gain control on the US regulates the amplification of returning echoes, exerting a pronounced influence on image brightness.

Increasing gain: Augments visibility of faint echoes, facilitating the detection of subtle hand structures.
Decreasing gain: Attenuates amplification, mitigating saturation in regions characterized by high echogenicity.

1.1.7 Doppler

The Doppler effect in US is a phenomenon related to the change in the frequency of sound waves as they encounter moving objects. In the context of medical imaging, including interventionism, it is particularly useful for assessing blood flow.

When sound waves encounter moving blood cells, the frequency of the waves changes. This change in frequency is detected and translated into color-coded images, showing the direction and speed of blood flow. The direction is determined by the way the flow is coming or leaving the probe: red approaching the probe and blue leaving the probe.

The usage of Doppler is useful in US-guided procedures for three reasons:

Arterial and venous mapping: Knowledge of the position of arteries and veins that are at risk during the procedure is essential. The use of Doppler enables a precise identification of the blood vessels, including possible variations in position and size. This mapping can influence the approach and type of surgery.
Real-time monitoring: Provides real-time information on blood flow dynamics during the procedure and helps practitioners make immediate adjustments in the position of the knife, enhancing the safety of interventions.
Post-intervention assessment: Enables post-intervention evaluation of blood flow to ensure no complications or injuries have occurred to vascular structures.

In summary, Doppler ultrasound is a valuable tool in US-guided procedures, as it provides dynamic information about vessel position, blood flow, and anatomical variability, thereby improving the safety of the procedure.

1.2 Ultrasound Anatomy

US-guided surgery relies on a thorough understanding of anatomy, emphasizing the crucial recognition of normal ultrasound patterns in common musculoskeletal structures [1, 2]

Tendons exhibit a distinct longitudinal fibrillar pattern, featuring alternating hyperechoic and hypoechoic lines. In the transverse axis, the renowned "salt and pepper" pattern emerges, showcasing a uniform distribution of hyperechoic granules amid hypoechoic elements.

Ligaments share similar characteristics, albeit with a less ordered pattern compared to tendons.

Muscles display a hypoechoic background corresponding to muscle fibers, with discernible hyperechoic lines representing connective tissue partitions. In the longitudinal axis, these partitions align parallelly, resembling a "bird's feather" architecture. In the transverse axis, the "starry sky" pattern emerges, consisting of alternating lines and hyperechoic points with a more disordered distribution.

Nerves have a more challenging evaluation, presenting fascicles as hypoechoic channels covered by perineurium in thick hyperechoic lines in the longitudinal axis, resembling the tendon's fibrillar pattern but with less organization, the so-called fascicular pattern. Cross-sectional views reveal a "blackberry-shaped" pattern, showcasing hypoechoic spots on a hyperechoic background.

Bone, reflecting the ultrasound beam almost entirely, generates a bright hyperechoic linear image with an acoustic shadow in-depth, limiting penetration.

Although ultrasound has limitations in joint evaluation, certain structures, such as cartilage, appear as a homogeneous hypoechoic line atop a hyperechoic line representing the subchondral bone. The joint capsule manifests as a thick hyperechoic line.

Vessels are visualized as hypoechoic images, with veins tending to be more voluminous and susceptible to collapse upon compression. Arteries, pulsatile in nature, possess thicker walls, providing increased resistance to compression.

1.3 Ultrasound Artifacts

Artifacts play a significant role in ultrasound US imaging, with particular emphasis on their relevance in US-guided surgery (Fig. 1.4). Noteworthy artifacts include:

1.3.1 Anisotropy

Anisotropy is observed in tissues with highly ordered and parallel internal architecture, such as tendons and ligaments. The appearance of these structures varies with the angle of the US beam. Tendons, for instance, may appear hyperechoic when the beam is perpendicular and gradually become more hypoechoic as the probe deviates from a 90° angle. This property allows clinicians to distinguish between different tissue types, a crucial factor during procedures like carpal tunnel releasing, where differentiation between the median nerve and adjacent finger flexor tendons is essential [3].

1.3.2 Shadowing

Shadowing occurs when the ultrasound beam is reflected by structures that impede its passage, resulting in an anechoic area deep from the interface. This can pose challenges in depth perception during surgery, especially when transitioning from soft tissue to bone or when evaluating abnormal calcifications within tendons [2].

1.3.3 Refractile Shadowing

Refractile shadowing is a specialized artifact observed when the ultrasound beam approaches a tissue interface at an oblique angle. Typically seen during A1 pulley releasing at the lateral margins of the tendon, this artifact occurs when the sound beam contacts the interface at a critical angle, beyond which refraction is no longer possible [3].

1.3.4 Reverberation

Commonly seen in US-guided surgery, reverberation artifact is induced by metallic instruments. It results from echoes produced when the ultrasound beam encounters interfaces with large differences in impedance within the body. These echoes take longer to return to the receiving crystals, leading to erroneous displays at greater tissue depths [3].

1.3.5 Comet Tail Artifact

A subtype of reverberation, the comet tail artifact is highly valuable in ultrasound-guided surgery. It consists of parallel hyperechoic bands that attenuate with increasing depth. The visualization of this artifact during invasive procedures ensures accurate identification of the observed structure, such as the knife or the material used in the procedure [3].

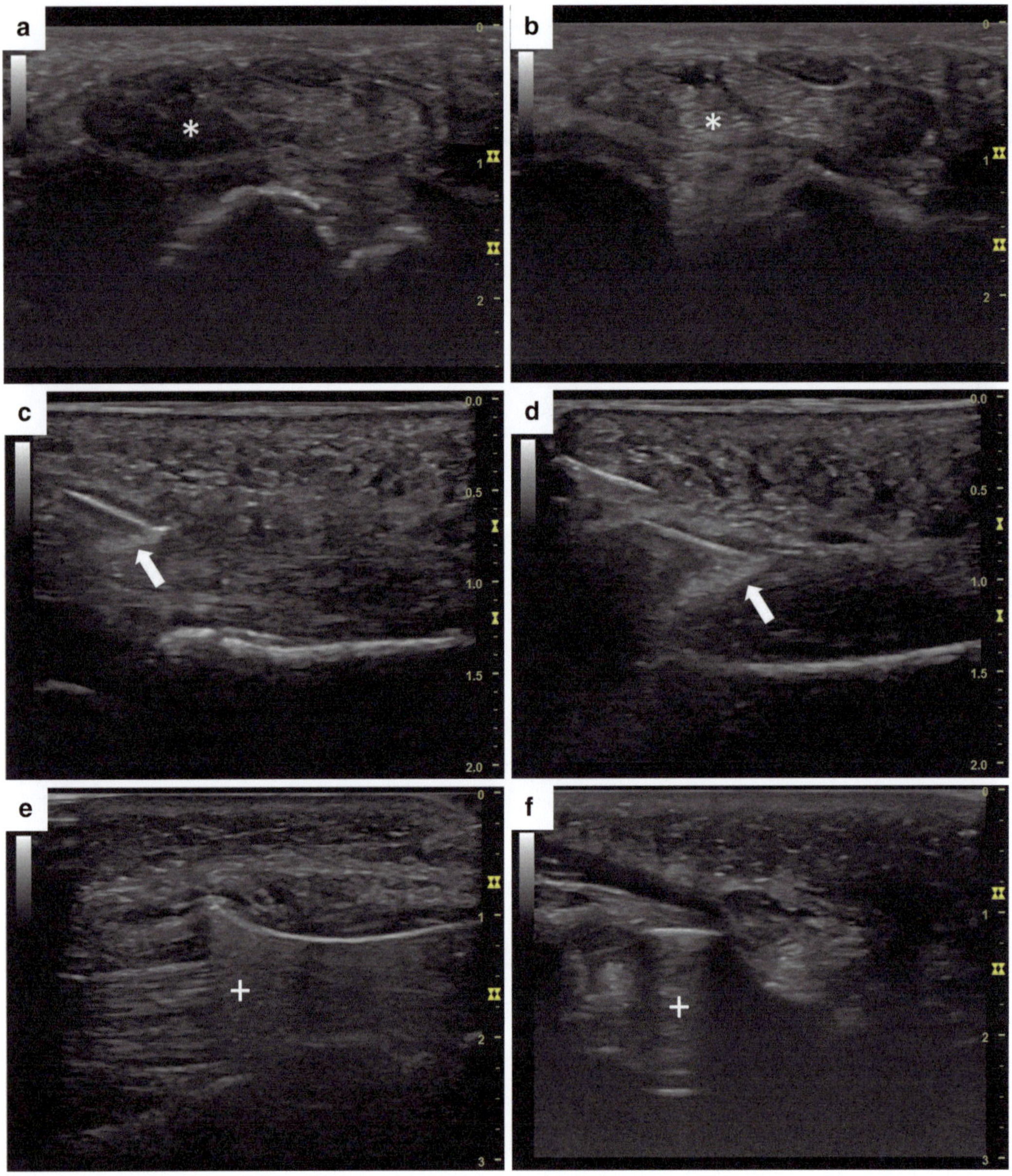

Fig. 1.4 (**a**, **b**) Anisotropy of the flexor tendons in the carpal tunnel. (**c**, **d**) Reverberation of a foreign body. (**e**, **f**) Comet tail artifact of a forceps during ultrasound-guided surgery

1.4 Ultrasound-Guided Technique

US-guided surgery necessitates meticulous technical considerations distinct from diagnostic ultrasound. Maintaining aseptic conditions is paramount, involving the encasement of the transducer in a sterile cover. However, this introduces challenges in handling [4].

1.4.1 Probe and Instrument Management

To address this, the nondominant hand is designated for transducer manipulation, while the dominant hand is allocated for the intricate maneuvering of surgical instruments like scalpels, mosquitoes, and needles. Precise transducer control is essential for proficient technical management, a critical factor in averting surgical complications.

Transducer control involves specific finger placement, where the thumb and second/third fingers orchestrate movements such as translation in both long and short axis, compression, rotation for plane adjustments, and oblique positioning during invasive procedures. Meanwhile, the fourth and fifth fingers serve as a stabilizing anchor, ensuring steadfast transducer grip and optimal visualization during the surgical intervention.

1.4.2 In-Plane Versus Out-of-Plane (Fig. 1.5)

Contemporary invasive procedures adopt a direct technique, characterized by continuous ultrasound visualization throughout the process, thereby mitigating potential complications [5]. Within this direct technique, two distinct approaches—in-plane and out-of-plane—dictate the alignment of surgical tools with the ultrasound transducer [2–6].

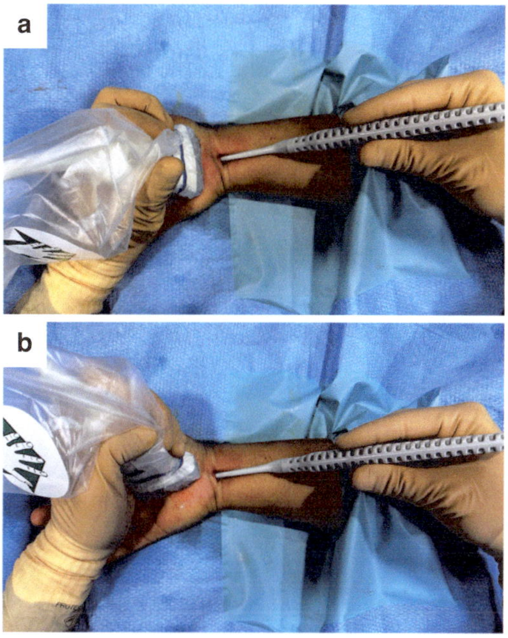

Fig. 1.5 (**a**) "Out-of-plane" technique, (**b**) "In-plane" technique

1.4.2.1 "In-Plane" Technique

Scalpel insertion aligns parallel to the transducer's long axis.

Employing the "stand-off oblique" technique enhances anisotropy, optimizing visibility of the scalpel.

This approach provides heightened control over the scalpel's depth and direction, minimizing the risk of inadvertent injury to adjacent anatomical structures.

1.4.2.2 "Out-of-Plane" Technique

Scalpel insertion occurs perpendicular to the transducer's long axis.

Adjusting the transducer's Tilt or Wag in the short axis optimizes visualization of the scalpel.

However, this technique offers a more limited field of view, restricting visibility to the segment immediately deepest to the transducer, thus heightening technical complexity and the risk of inadvertent injury.

In the out-of-plane technique, the "Walk down" method is imperative. This entails a strategic approach involving iterative scalpel withdrawal and advancement, allowing precise navigation until the target area is reached. This minimizes the risk of penetrating too deeply or extending beyond the defined ultrasound plane.

Proficiency in both in-plane and out-of-plane techniques is indispensable for successful ultrasound-guided surgery. Mastery of these methodologies ensures precise scalpel positioning, contributing to optimal procedural outcomes and patient safety.

Take-Home Message

Ultrasound machines need a prefect setup to be able to realize ultrasound assessment and ultrasound guidance gesture.

Setup include:

Frequency, general gain, depth and focus.

It is necessary to know how to setup all these items before starting using ultrasound.

Artifacts:

Must be known to understand the ultrasound image, such as anisotropy, comet tail, and shadow cone.

These artifacts are due to the interaction of the anatomical structures and the ultrasound waves.

Ultrasound-guided procedure planification:

When ultrasound gestures are programmed, the operator should know.

Needs for "out-of-plane" or "in-plane" view of the anatomical structure. How to cover the probe and to ensure the sterility field.

Specific instruments that are needed and should be used to realize ultrasound guidance gesture.

References

1. Smith J, Finnoff JT. Diagnostic and interventional musculoskeletal ultrasound: part 2. Clinical applications. PM R. 2009;1(2):162–77.
2. Herbert Stevenson J. Tissue scanning. In: Daniels JM, Dexter WW, editors. Basics of musculoskeletal ultrasound; 2013. p. 15–27.
3. Maxwell MD, Weber NH, Chimes GP. Ultrasound physics for interventional procedures. In: Malanga G, Mautner K, editors. Atlas of ultrasound-guide muskuloskeletal injections. Mc Graw Hill Education; 2014. p. 6–13.
4. Smith J, Finnoff JT. Diagnostic and interventional musculoskeletal ultrasound: part 1. Fundamentals. PM R. 2009;1(1):64–75.
5. Del Cura JL, Zabala R, Corta I. US-guided interventional procedures: what a radiologist needs to know. Radiologia. 2010;52(3):198–207.
6. Visco CJ. Introduction to interventional ultrasound. In: Malanga G, Mautner K, editors. Atlas of ultrasound-guide muskuloskeletal injections. Mc Graw Hill Education; 2014. p. 2–5.

What Setting for Ultrasound-Guided Surgery

2

Bernáldez Domínguez

2.1 Introduction

Minimally invasive surgery (MI) has become a fundamental approach in sports traumatology, allowing patients a faster recovery and fewer postoperative complications. One of the key elements in this type of procedure is ultrasound-guided surgery [1], allowing unprecedented precision (Fig. 2.1). In this article, we will explore the essential instruments used in ultrasound-guided surgery, highlighting their accessibility, their low economic cost, and their application in various areas and tissues of the musculoskeletal system, as well as the latest developments in this type of instrumentation.

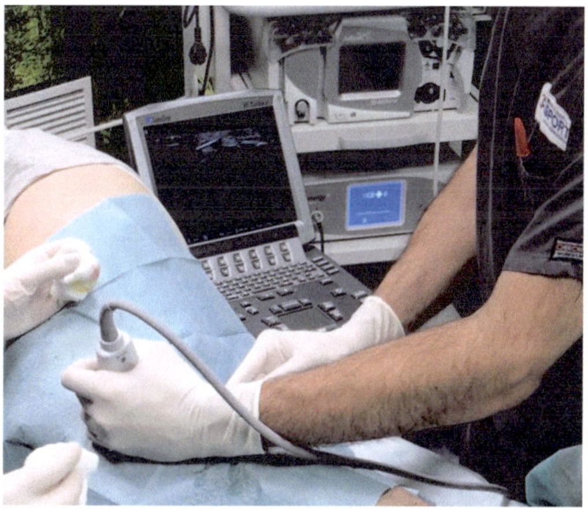

Fig. 2.1 Ultrasound-guided surgery of the iliotibial band

B. Domínguez (✉)
Department of Orthopedic Surgery and Sports Traumatology, Ultrasound-guided Interventionism and Orthobiology Unit, SportMe Medical Center and OrtobioSevilla (Seville), Seville, Spain

O. Marès et al. (eds.), *Ultrasound-Guided Limb Surgery*,
https://doi.org/10.1007/978-3-031-88679-9_2

2.2 Basic Instruments for Ultrasound-Guided Surgery

Ultrasound-guided surgery is based on the use of ultrasound equipment to visualize anatomical structures in real time. Although ultrasound equipment can vary in terms of features and prices, the instrumentation required to perform these procedures is usually simple and affordable [2] (Fig. 2.2). Here are the most essential elements:

2.2.1 Ultrasound Probe

The ultrasound probe is the main tool in ultrasound-guided surgery. It provides real-time images that allow the surgeon to visualize anatomical structures and guide surgery precisely.

Linear probe: Used for the evaluation of superficial structures, such as muscles, tendons, ligaments, nerves, and joints. It provides high-resolution images [3].

Convex probe: Useful for examining deeper structures in the body, especially the hip and spine. It can also be used for studies of other soft tissues in the musculoskeletal system.

Microconvex probe: Similar to the convex probe, but with a smaller, curved design, it is suitable for evaluating anatomical superficial structures and can be especially useful in areas with limited space.

Stick probe: They are high-frequency probes and are used to obtain detailed images of superficial structures, such as tendons and ligaments. They offer exceptional resolution.

2.2.2 Needles

The needles used in ultrasound-guided surgery are essential for the different gestures that we will perform such as microperforations [4], aspiration of fluids, injection of medications, tears, or even the insertion of devices such as sutures or threads. The needles should be thin enough to minimize damage to surrounding tissues (Fig. 2.3).

There are special needles with a "mini-scalpel" bevel end such as the "Admix Needles" allowing you to tear or cut tissue.

There are also needles with a small hole at the tip that allows suture threads to be transported, ideal for tendon sutures. Some incorporate a handle, which makes it easier to perform the technique.

2.2.3 Scalpel Blades

Thin, sharp scalpel blades are used to make minimal incisions in the skin or soft tissue. This helps minimize trauma and recovery time. There are

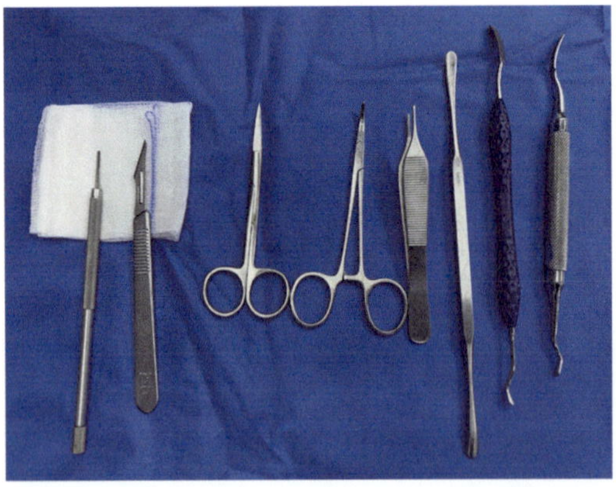

Fig. 2.2 Basic instrumentation

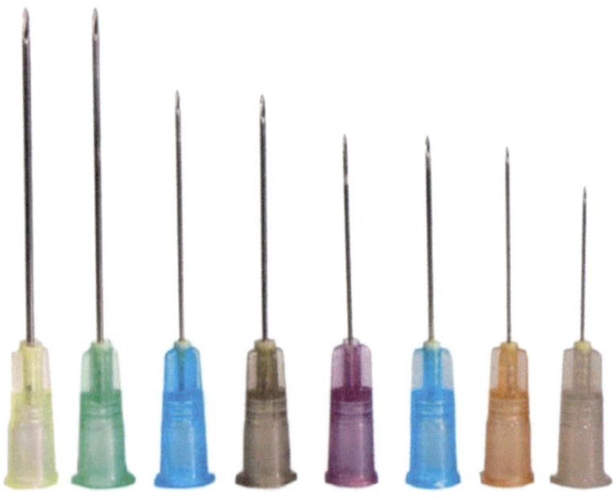

Fig. 2.3 Needles used in ultrasound-guided surgery

different sizes, models, and designs on the market. Being metallic makes it much easier to see on the ultrasound screen. Percutaneous minimally invasive surgery (MIS) of the foot has greatly facilitated the use of ultrasound-assisted surgery (Fig. 2.4). Specific scalpels have even been designed for some specific surgeries such as carpal tunnel release.

2.2.4 Basic Instruments

Scissors: Fine-tipped scissors are useful for making precise cuts in tissues, such as ligaments or tendons, when necessary.

Mosquitoes or tweezers: These forceps are essential for grasping, manipulating, and holding tissues during surgery.

Specific devices: In some cases, specific devices designed for pathologies such as carpal tunnel syndrome [1], cubital tunnel syndrome, and medial gastrocnemius release may be used.

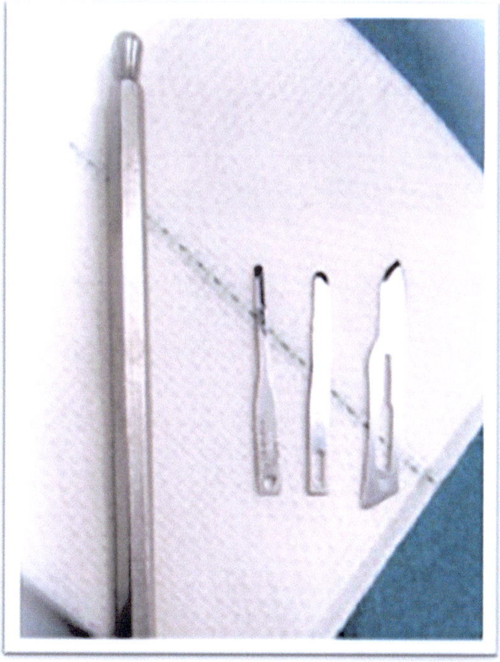

Fig. 2.4 Scalpels used in ultrasound-guided surgery

2.3 Specific Instruments for Hand Surgery

In sports trauma, hand and wrist injuries are common. Minimally invasive ultrasound-guided surgery has become especially valuable in this area [5–9]. To address hand injuries, additional instruments may be used, such as:

Injection needles: Fine injection needles are essential for administering local anesthesia, corticosteroids, PRP, etc. to specific areas of the hand, such as joints or tendons.

Hooks: These instruments allow the exploration and manipulation of anatomical structures in narrow spaces, such as the tendon canals of the hand and opening of retinaculum (Fig. 2.5).

Neurovascular protective devices: Without a doubt, the biggest complication of this type of surgery is neurovascular injury, for example, damaging the median nerve in carpal tunnel syndrome surgery. Therefore, it is important to use protective devices to avoid this complication (Fig. 2.6).

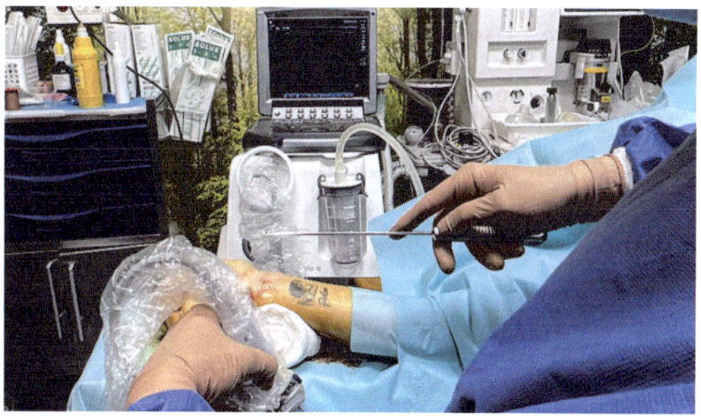

Fig. 2.5 Hook devices for US-guided surgery

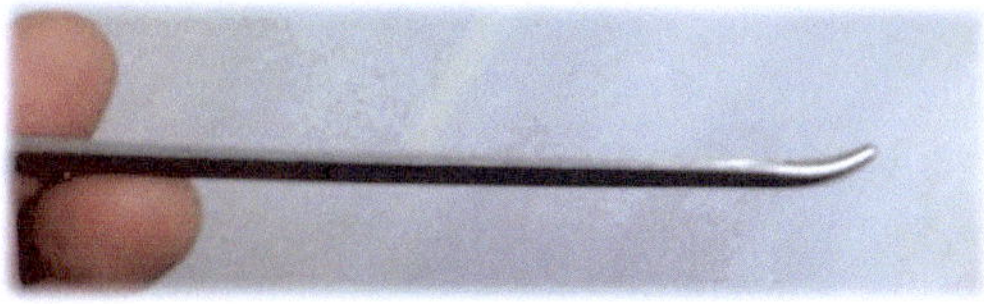

Fig. 2.6 Protective sleeve for neurovascular structures

Mini-scalpels: These are useful for ensuring a precise cut (e.g., in a fibrous cord in Dupuytren's disease), in the desired location, minimizing the risk of further injury.

Fixation devices: In the repair of tendons or ligaments in the hand, minimally invasive fixation devices, such as suture anchors, can be used to ensure solid fixation.

Arthroscopic shaver: Arthroscopic surgery can be combined with ultrasound-guided surgery in what we have called "echo-arthroscopic surgery" and for this it is essential to use an arthroscopic shaver to proceed with tissue resection. One of the most common indications is wrist ganglions.

2.4 Ultrasound Therapy Devices

In recent times, there have been significant advances in the treatment of tendinopathies using ultrasound devices [10]. These devices enable high-intensity focused ultrasound (HIFU) therapy or extracorporeal shockwave therapy (ESWT) to address soft tissue injuries such as tendons.

HIFU therapy [11] uses focused ultrasound to generate heat in a specific area of tissue. This heat dries out degenerative tissue and can stimulate tendon repair and reduce inflammation. On the other hand, ESWT therapy involves the application of shockwaves through the skin to stimulate tissue regeneration and reduce pain [12]. Both approaches are minimally invasive and offer an alternative to traditional surgery in the treatment of tendinopathies.

2.5 Where the Future Is Going

Since the appearance of small micro-cameras placed in small caliber needles, we are able to combine real images with ultrasounds, all in a single platform or tablet-type screen, which allows a mobility and accessibility never seen before, ideal to introduce into the operating room.

2.5.1 Advantages

- The micro-endoscope allows for percutaneous procedures with less scarring and lower post-operative risks.
- The combination of the two technologies makes it possible to monitor patients more easily thanks to the recording ability of the procedures (ultrasound guided or endoscopic).
- It increases the safety of procedures by improving the accuracy of approaches.
- Improves diagnostic capability without resorting to ionized imaging technologies.
- Faster and more comfortable procedures for the patient increase postoperative satisfaction.
- The color image from the HD camera, displayed next to the ultrasound image, makes it easier to visualize and accurately explore body structures.

A combination of mini-ultra devices that allows us to view dynamic images (including joint images) to diagnose joint injuries with clarity and confidence, in real time. They are compact, lightweight, and easily transportable and with high-quality images.

2.6 Author's Experience

Ultrasound-assisted surgery requires a significant learning curve, since it combines knowledge of both ultrasound management and surgical techniques, but for an experienced orthopedic surgeon, they are minimally invasive, simple techniques, with reproducible gestures, since they are normally surgeries to release tendon structures or fascia. With precise instruments, it will help us to perform the technique properly and normally without complications. Percutaneous tendon suturing also plays an important role.

Perhaps the most dedicated part is locating the neurovascular structures so as not to damage

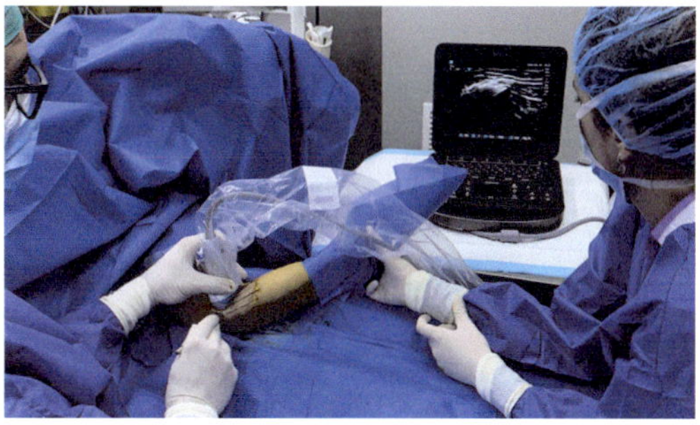

Fig. 2.7 Epitrocleitis ultrasound-guided surgery

them. We have performed more than 80 ultrasound-guided surgeries (Fig. 2.7) with a very satisfactory balance, good results for patients, and no complications to highlight; however, it is a technique that must continue to be implemented, and practical courses on cadavers is one of the most important tools to disseminate knowledge.

2.7 Conclusions

Ultrasound-guided minimally invasive surgery has revolutionized sports traumatology by providing unprecedented precision and faster recovery for patients [13]. The instrumentation used in these procedures is affordable and relatively straightforward, making it an attractive option for surgeons. In this article, we have described the most frequently used instruments and even the new features for the future.

In addition, in the treatment of tendinopathies, ultrasound devices have opened up new possibilities for the nonsurgical approach to soft tissue injuries [14].

The future of sports traumatology lies in the constant evolution of these minimally invasive techniques, which continue to improve patients' quality of life and reduce recovery time. The combination of high-quality instrumentation and state-of-the-art technology promises exciting breakthroughs in this ever-growing area.

References

1. Bernáldez Domínguez P, Dallo Lazzarini I. State-of-the-art in ultrasound-guided surgery: Concept, planning, instruments, classifications, indications, and literature review. J Regener Sci. 2022;2(1):16.
2. Bernáldez Domínguez P. The ultrasound: the stethoscope of the traumatologist: diagnostic and therapeutic utility. Rev Traum Ort. 2017;34:17–26.
3. Bernáldez Domínguez P. The third hand. Rev S Traum Ort. 2019;36(2/4):56–7.
4. Bernáldez Domínguez P. Ultrasound-guided therapies (EG) in traumatology: seeing what we do and how we treat it. Rev SLAOT. 2019;4(2)
5. Rojo-Manaute JM, Capa-Grasa A, Chana-Rodríguez F, Perez-Mañanes R, Rodriguez-Maruri G, Sanz-Ruiz P, et al. Ultra-minimally invasive ultrasound-guided carpal tunnel release: a randomized clinical trial. J Ultrasound Med. 2016;35:1149–57.
6. Buncke G, McCormack B, Bodor M. Ultrasound-guided carpal tunnel release using the manos CTR system. Microsurgery. 2013;33:362–6.
7. De la Fuente J, Miguel-Perez MI, Balius R, Guerrero V, Michaud J, Bong D. Minimally invasive ultrasound-guided carpal tunnel release: a cadaver study. J Clin Ultrasound. 2013;41:101–7.
8. Lecoq B, Hanouz N, Vielpeau C, Marcelli C. Ultrasound-guided percutaneous surgery for carpal tunnel syndrome: a cadaver study. Joint Bone Spine. 2011;78:516–8.
9. Smith J, Rizzo M, Lai JK. Sonographically guided percutaneous first annular pulley release: cadaveric safety study of needle and knife techniques. J Ultrasound Med. 2010;29:1531–42.
10. Vajapey S, Ghenbot S, Baria MR, Magnussen RA, Vasileff WK. Utility of percutaneous ultrasonic Tenotomy for tendinopathies: a systematic review. Sports Health. 2021;13(3):258–64.
11. Mihcin S, Melzer A. Principles of focused ultrasound. Minim Invasive Ther Allied Technol. 2018;27(1):41–50.
12. Schroeder AN, Tenforde AS, Jelsing EJ. Extracorporeal shockwave therapy in the management of sports medicine injuries. Curr Sports Med Rep. 2021;20(6):298–305.
13. Sconfienza LM, Adriaensen M, Albano D, Alcalá-Galiano A, Allen G, Gómez MB, et al. Clinical indications for image-guided interventional procedures in the musculoskeletal system: a Delphi-based consensus paper from the European society of musculoskeletal radiology (ESSR)-part V, knee. Eur Radiol. 2022;32(3):1438–47.
14. Smith J, Sellon JL. Interventional musculoskeletal ultrasound in sports medicine: current concepts and evidence. Curr Sports Med Rep. 2019;18(6):217–22.

How to Draw a Sterile Probe

3

Francisco Javier Ferreira

3.1 Introduction

Ultrasound-guided procedures have become a standard practice in various medical fields due to their precision and effectiveness. When performing ultrasound-guided interventions, maintaining sterility is crucial to prevent infections and ensure patient safety.

Ultrasound probes are reusable instruments, which can be used to perform several examinations and procedure per day, including single-shot injections and ultrasound-guided surgery. Because of their reusable nature, they are ideal vectors for cross contamination if not protected and cleaned correctly. Using a sterile probe for ultrasound-guided musculoskeletal procedures involves wiping the probe with a disinfection wipe and using a sterile gel [1].

Concerns about the possibility of infection spread by *ultrasound probes* have increased as procedures using *ultrasound* become more popular. Several studies have suggested various preparation methods ranging from the use of simple dry nonsterile towels to the use of commercially available single-use *sterile probe* covers [2].

Depending on the procedure to be performed, we can use different types of covers for our transducer, including the probe or the complete transducer including its cable.

Studies have shown that the risk of infection transmission post ultrasound-guided procedures, where sterile single-use covers are used, is low [3].

It is also important to clean the transducer used in an invasive procedure with an appropriate disinfectant before and after it.

3.2 Ultrasound Probe Sterilization Protocol

After cleaning the probe of visible traces of gel or dirt, it should be disinfected using an appropriate disinfectant after each patient to ensure proper sterilization. Following the disinfection process is crucial to prevent the spread of infections. The products recommended by manufacturers for cleaning ultrasound equipment, including probes, usually have quaternary ammonium in their composition.

Although the above is true, it is necessary to distinguish between endocavitary ultrasound procedures such as those performed through the esophagus or vagina, which are much more contaminating, and external probes such as those performed in musculoskeletal ultrasound. In the latter case, cleaning the probe with a dry wipe; a conventional disinfectant, such as chlorhexidine; or soapy water is enough to significantly reduce

F. J. Ferreira (✉)
Hospital Universitario San Rafael, Madrid, Spain

International Chair of Musculoskeletal Ultrasound. UCAM, Murcia, Spain
e-mail: javierferreira@drjavierferreira.com

O. Marès et al. (eds.), *Ultrasound-Guided Limb Surgery*,
https://doi.org/10.1007/978-3-031-88679-9_3

the contamination of the probe. It is important, since we are going to carry out this process many times throughout the life of our probe, not to use aggressive products that can damage the plastic covers, especially the membrane, of the probe.

In all ultrasound-guided procedures, sterile gloves will be used by the medical staff who will perform the procedure. The need for surgical gowns and large sterile fields is not yet protocolized in many countries.

Depending on the ultrasound-guided procedure we perform, the asepsis needs for the probe or the hole transducer are different:

3.2.1 Ultrasound-Guided Injections

In these cases, after properly disinfecting the skin of the area where we will perform the puncture, and having disinfected the probe, we will proceed to cover the probe, after applying nonsterile gel to the membrane, with a suitable sterile cover (Fig. 3.1), with no need for the sterile coverage of the entire transducer [1]. If we don't have a sterile cover for the probe or it is too big for the probe used (i.e., hockey stick probe), we can use a sterile digit of a surgical glove and a sterile rubber band to keep it in place (Fig. 3.2).

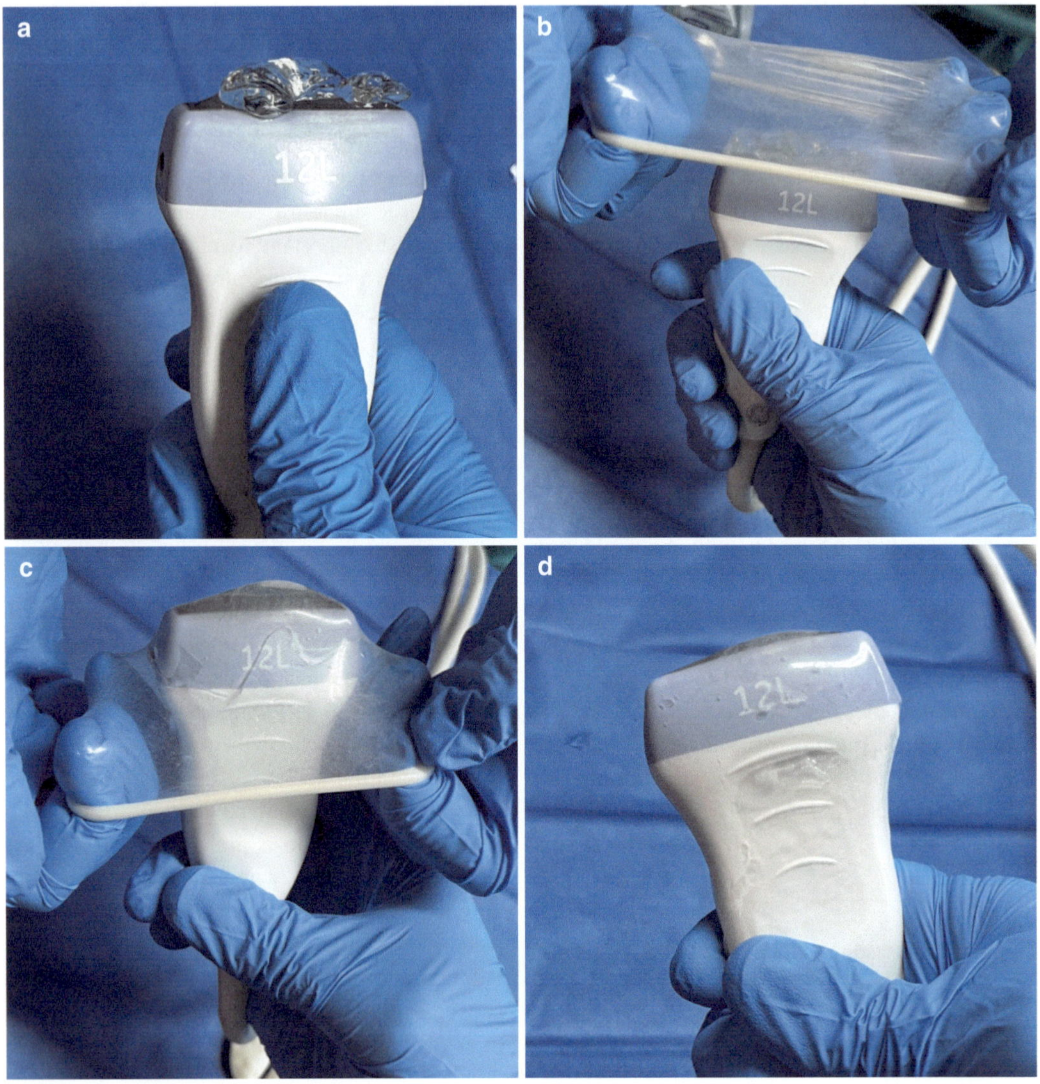

Fig. 3.1 Covering the probe with a sterile cover suitable for injections. (**a**) Gel application over the membrane. (**b**, **c**) application of the cover. (**d**) Probe ready

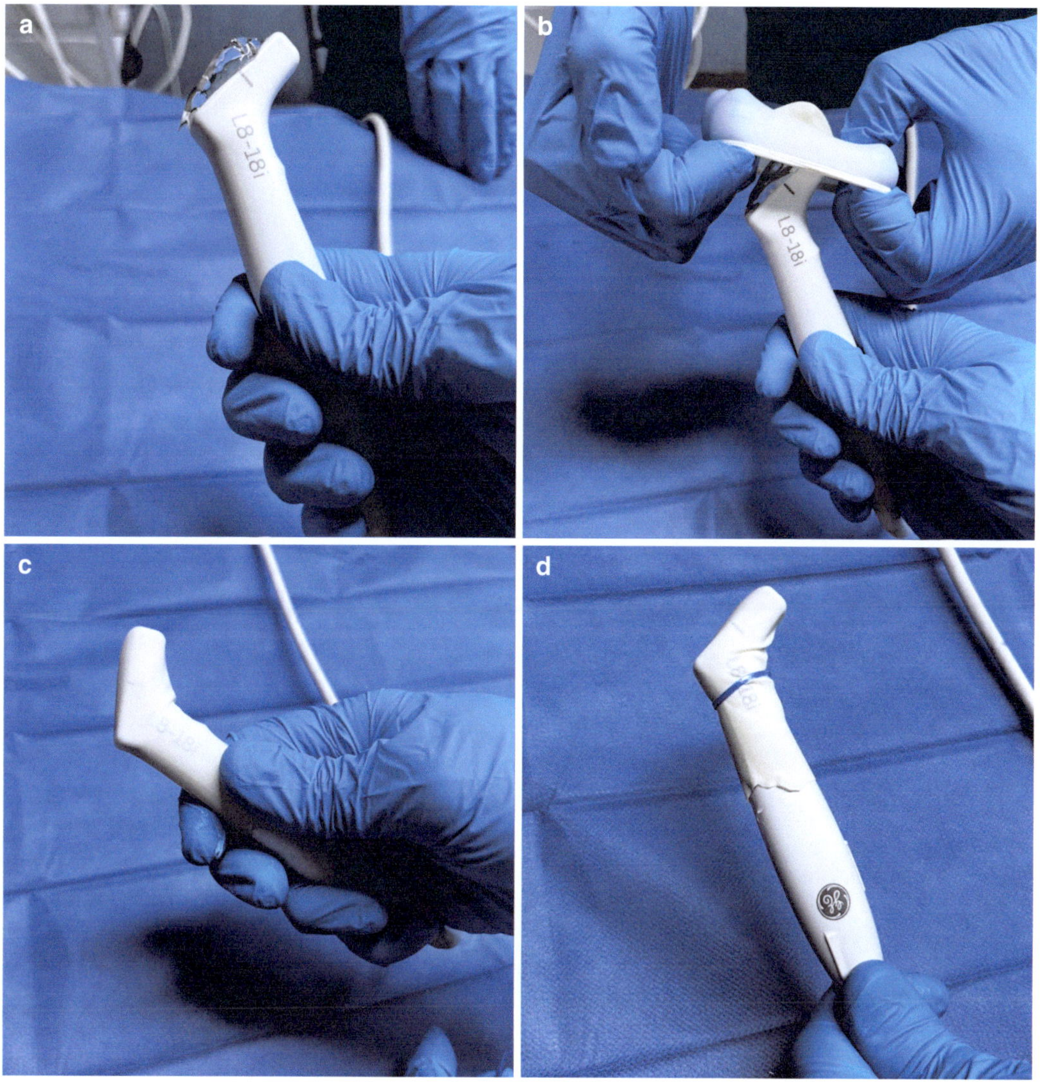

Fig. 3.2 Covering "hockey-stick" probe. (**a**) Gel application over the membrane. (**b**, **c**) Covering the distal part of the probe with a sterile finger glove. (**d**) Applying a sterile rubber band

We will use sterile gel as conductive fluid, which is usually supplied in individual packages or a disinfectant liquid or gel such as Betadine gel®.

3.2.2 Ultrasound-Guided Surgery

In ultrasound-guided surgical procedures, once the surgical team is dressed if we do an operating room procedure or put on sterile gloves when performing an office-based procedure, we proceed to do a correct skin disinfection of the area to be treated with an antiseptic solution containing isopropyl alcohol, povidone iodine and/or chlorhexidine gluconate, and then we place a sterile field with drapes that delimit the surgical area we are about to treat. Afterwards we will use a sterile cover of the entire transducer, including the cable [4]. There are specific transducer covers on the market, although arthroscopy camara covers can also be used by adding a sterile transparent dressing such as Tegaderm ® (Fig. 3.3). A circulating nurse holds the probe, and the surgical team

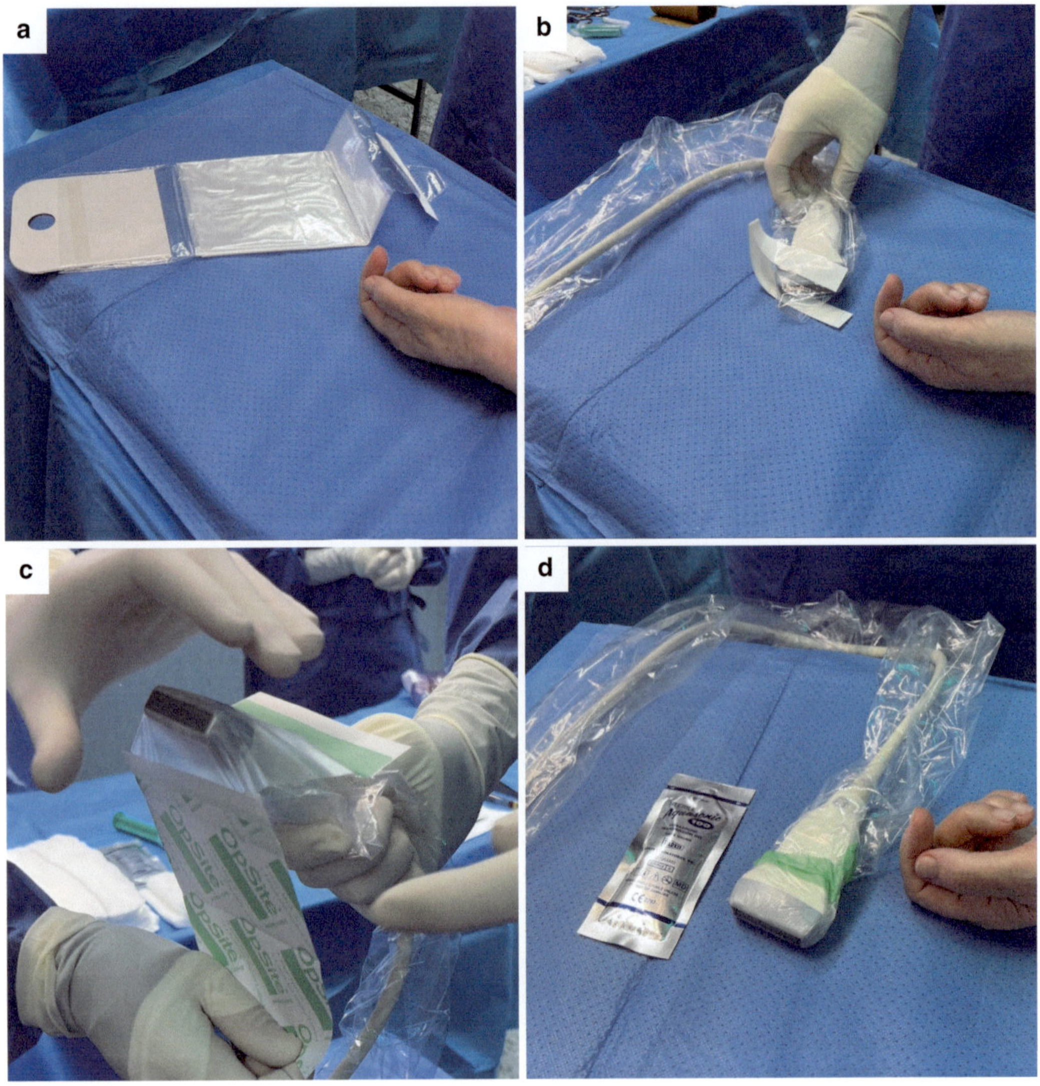

Fig. 3.3 Draping the transducer for an ultrasound-guided surgery. (**a**) Conventional sterile arthroscopic camera cover. (**b**) Transducer (probe + cable) introduced inside the cover. (**c**) Applying an sterile transparent waterproof dressing (no gel is needed in this step). (**d**) Sterile transducer and gel

encases the transducer. In the case of specific covers, we must previously cover the membrane of the area with gel, while in the case of using transparent dressings, these are applied directly to the membrane. When performing scanning during the procedure, we will always apply sterile gel over the patient's skin as a conductive fluid.

Bibliography

1. Bang S, Lee H, Kim ED. Assessment of condoms for probe preparation method for ultrasound-guided musculoskeletal injections: a prospective, randomized non-inferiority trial. Med Biol Sci Eng. 2023;6:20–5.
2. Lorentzen T, et al. EFSUMB guidelines on Interventional Ultrasound (INVUS), part I. Ultraschall Med. 2015;36:E3–E16.
3. Westerway SC, Basseal JM. The ultrasound unit and infection control—are we on the right track? Ultrasound. 2017;25:53–7.
4. Lopez SA, et al. Design, prototyping, and evaluation of a collapsible device for single-operator sheathing of ultrasound probes. Mech Sci. 2014;5:7–13.

Part II

Hand

4 Ultrasound-Guided Percutaneous Surgical Technique for Trigger Finger Release

Michiel Cromheecke

4.1 Introduction

Trigger finger, also known as stenosing tenovaginitis, is a prevalent inflammatory disorder affecting the A1 pulleys of the fingers, frequently causing hand discomfort and pain [1]. The lifetime risk is estimated to be around 2.6% [2]. This condition is marked by finger locking and localized pain, stemming from the stenosing tenovaginitis at the A1 pulley. Notable thickening of both the A1 pulley and the flexor tendon has been observed in this condition [2].

The main goal of surgical treatment for the trigger finger is to release the A1 pulley, which reduces friction and the snapping of the flexor tendon. This leads to a decrease in synovitis and inflammation, ultimately alleviating pain.

Although open A1 pulley release remains the conventional gold standard, there is an increasing shift toward minimally invasive percutaneous approaches. These methods vary from blind percutaneous needle techniques to more sophisticated procedures using hook knives, with some incorporating ultrasound guidance for enhanced precision. First introduced by Lorthioir in 1958, the percutaneous release technique has become increasingly popular owing to its simplicity, reduced pain and recovery time, absence of a painful scar on the palm, and lower costs [3, 4]. Initially, these procedures primarily utilized hypodermic needles. Research indicates high success rates in symptom resolution, low recurrence, and minimal complications with percutaneous techniques, although concerns persist regarding the potential for incomplete releases and superficial tendon injuries when employing needle techniques [3].

This chapter introduces an innovative ultrasound-guided percutaneous method that utilizes a minimally invasive surgical knife. The "simplicity" of this technique ensures consistent complete release while minimizing complications. This is well aided by the real-time visualization ultrasound guidance.

The shift from conventional open surgical methods to minimally invasive percutaneous and ultrasound-assisted techniques mark a significant advancement in treating trigger fingers. These methods not only are effective in relieving symptoms but also notably cut down on costs and surgery time, and they reduce potential risks. Additionally, they offer the benefit of a shorter postoperative recovery period.

4.2 Diagnosis

Trigger finger diagnosis is primarily clinical. Patients might report a painless clicking or snapping sensation in the finger during flexion extension. This clicking can gradually become

M. Cromheecke (✉)
Hand, Wrist and Shoulder Surgery, AZ Maria Middelares, Ghent, Belgium

O. Marès et al. (eds.), *Ultrasound-Guided Limb Surgery*,
https://doi.org/10.1007/978-3-031-88679-9_4

painful. The discomfort and mechanical symptoms are often localized at the A1 pulley, although can be referred to as the metacarpophalangeal (MCP) or proximal interphalangeal (PIP) joints [5].

Patients may also experience increased stiffness, especially in the morning, and a progressive loss of full flexion and/or extension in the affected finger, sometimes without the classic catching and locking. In most individuals, a palpable nodule due to intratendinous swelling can be detected in the palmar A1 area. This nodule is often tender to the touch and can contribute to the feeling of stiffness or swelling, particularly noticeable in the morning. Some patients even report waking up with the digit locked in a bent position, which gradually loosens throughout the day.

With further deterioration, the affected finger may become locked in a flexed position, requiring manual manipulation to extend it fully. This locking occurs because the flexor mechanisms in the finger are usually strong enough to push through the tight and narrowed retinacular sheath, whereas the extensor mechanisms are less capable. In advanced stages, patients may inadvertently develop secondary PIP joint contractures and increased stiffness in the digit. A commonly used classification of trigger finger severity is Green's classification (Table 4.1).

In addition to these clinical signs, ultrasonography can support the diagnosis, which is particularly useful in visualizing the pathology at the tendon-pulley interface. This imaging modality can confirm the diagnosis, especially in cases where the clinical presentation is ambiguous or when other hand pathologies need to be ruled out [1].

4.3 Treatment Options

Trigger finger leads doctors and patients to seek various treatment options. Common first-line treatment includes the use of occupational therapy, splinting, and corticosteroid injections. Steroid injections have shown effectiveness in between 45% and 80%. However, their effectiveness is less pronounced in diabetic patients, with success rates reported between 32% and 66% [1, 6]. Recurrency rate is also thought to be higher in diabetic patients, though this is opposed by others [7]. Newport et al. reported improvement in only 23% of the patients who needed a second injection and 5% in those needing a third injection [6]. These injections are particularly beneficial in improving grip strength, pain, and frequency of triggering events, though their efficacy tends to wane with a recurrence rate of 61% at a mean time of 312 days [8]. When conservative interventions fail, surgical options are considered. Open surgical release of the A1 pulley, the benchmark operation for TF, has success rates reported between 90% and 100%. Percutaneous A1 pulley release is an emerging alternative with growing support in the literature. It is a safe and effective method and literature shows no additional complications are to be expected [9, 10] compared to open surgery. Despite these findings, surgeons hesitate to implement these new techniques in their daily practice. Additionally, percutaneous techniques demand a learning curve. It's noted that many hand surgery training programs do not routinely offer exposure to percutaneous trigger finger release, suggesting a need for additional education for surgeons not yet skilled in this technique.

Table 4.1 Green classification for trigger finger

Green classification		
Grade		Clinical feature
I (pretrigger)		Pain or tenderness over the A1 pulley. Reporting history of catching or locking.
II (active)		Demonstrable catching on physical examination with preserved active extension.
III (passive)	IIIA	Locking of the finger requiring passive extension.
	IIIB	Impossibility of active flexion of the finger.
IV (contracture)		Demonstrable locking of the finger with a flexion contracture of the PIP joint.

Source: Wolfe SW: Tendinopathy, in Wolfe SW, Hotchkiss RN, Pederson WC, Kozin SH, Cohen MS, Eds.: Green's Operative Hand Surgery, seventh Edition, Philadelphia: Elsevier, 2017; pp. 1903–1925.

4.4 Personal Technique

4.4.1 Indications and Contraindications

This technique is indicated for the release of the long digits (index, middle finger, ring finger, little finger). It should be noted that the thumb is better released using a retrograde technique. All grades of trigger fingers can be treated using this technique, but in cases of preexisting extension deficits of the proximal interphalangeal joint (PIP), these are often not fully corrected after the release of the A1 pulley. This is in accordance with the results of classical open release. In these cases, we feel that resection of the ulnar slip of the superficial flexor tendon can be considered as described by Le Viet et al. [11].

4.4.2 Setup

The surgery is best performed under local anesthesia or distal nerve block to examine the active motion of the fingers and confirm the alleviation of triggering symptoms.

In our setup, we use a wide-awake local anesthesia no tourniquet (WALANT). A 10 ml of 1% lidocaine with 1:100.000 epinephrine is locally instilled just proximal to the A1 pulley in the subcutaneous soft tissue. The arm can be draped in a sterile setup using a draping with a hole. The surgeon is wearing sterile clothing and gloves. The ultrasound probe is covered with sterile gel and a sterile cover to be used in the surgical zone. This surgery can be performed in an office or operation room setting. The necessary instruments for this procedure are limited. A possible setup for this procedure can be seen in Fig. 4.1.

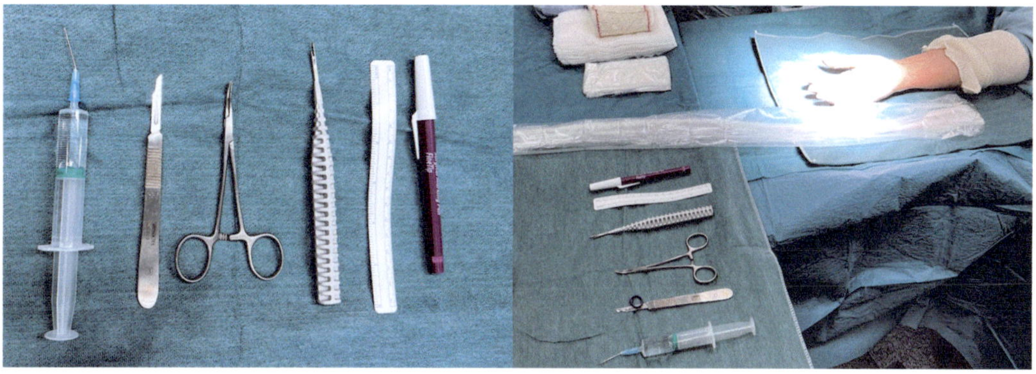

Fig. 4.1 Setup needed for ultrasound-guided trigger finger release. A minimal amount of instruments is needed. A single use knife can be used. This way sterilization costs can be reduced

4.5 Surgical Anatomy

In the context of minimally invasive percutaneous methods, a thorough understanding of surgical anatomy is crucial. Hence, precise knowledge about the A1 pulley's location and the flexor tendon is imperative. Figure 4.2 illustrates the path of the flexor tendons and marks the proximal edge of the A1 pulley. A reliable method to identify the proximal edge of the A1 pulley was proposed by Fiorini et al. in 2011 [12]. This involves measuring the distance from the digital palmar to the proximal interphalangeal crease, providing a consistent means to locate the A1 pulley's proximal edge, which is found to be nearly the same distance proximal from the digital palmar crease.

The distal border of the A1 pulley can be seen using ultrasound. An anatomical landmark for this point was described by Jurbala et al. [13]. The distal border of the pulley can consistently be found at the bony peak of the proximal phalanx. This is identified as the bony ridge between the metaphysis and diaphysis of the proximal phalanx (Fig. 4.3).

When performing a release, it is best to mark the direction of the flexor tendons. Keep in mind that all flexor tendons converge toward the outlet of the carpal tunnel. We advise verifying your markings and the direction using ultrasound, especially for the index and little finger.

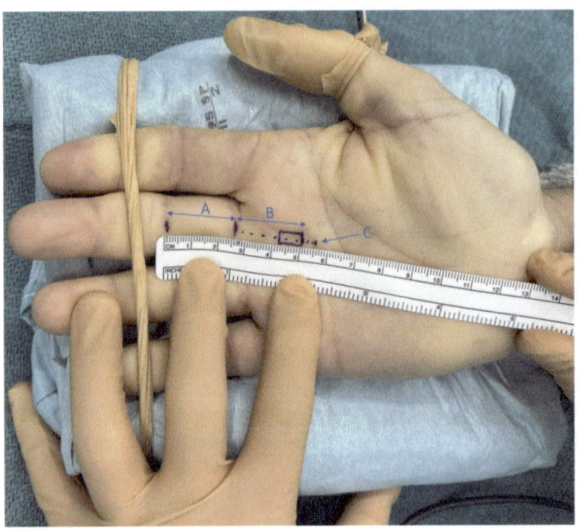

Fig. 4.2 Topographic anatomy and anatomic landmarks of the A1 flexor tendon pulley and marking method for incision. Distance (**a**) is defined as the distance between the palmodigital crease and the proximal interphalangeal crease. This equals distance (**b**), at which point the proximal edge of the A1 pulley can be found. A good point for incision can be found at about 0.5 cm proximal to this edge (**c**). Note that all tendons converge in the direction of the carpal tunnel

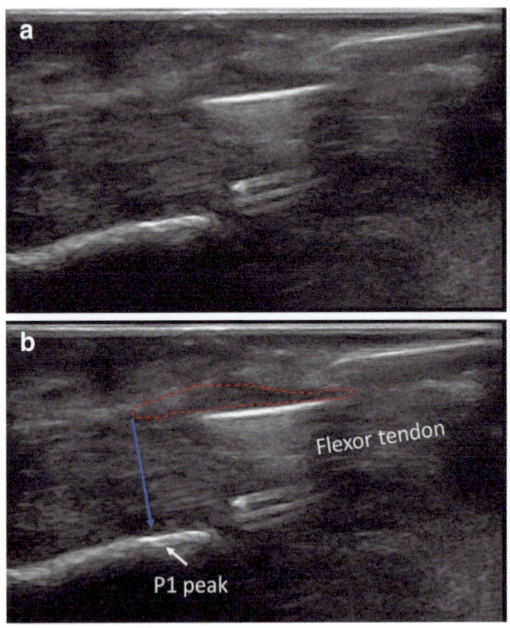

Fig. 4.3 (**a**) Illustration of the cutting mechanism of the surgical knife. (**b**) Marking of the A1 pulley (red dotted line). The distal edge of the A1 pulley can be found at same level as the "P1 peak." This is identified as the bony ridge between the metaphysis and diaphysis of the proximal phalanx

4.6 Surgical Technique

The initial step involves accurately marking the path of the flexor tendon in the hand's palm and identifying the A1 pulley's proximal edge, as described earlier (Fig. 4.2). This is confirmed by feeling the metacarpal head beneath the A1 pulley and ultrasound verification. After identifying these anatomical landmarks, a minor incision, approximately 5 mm proximal to the A1 pulley's edge, is created. Typically, this incision is positioned at the proximal palmar crease for the index finger and at the distal palmar crease for the middle, ring, and little fingers. Subsequently, a curved mosquito forceps is gently inserted between the flexor tendon and the A1 pulley without harming adjacent critical structures (Fig. 4.4). Upon successful insertion of the forceps under the A1 pulley, a resistance of the pulley is felt against skin approximation; this can later be used as an indication to confirm complete surgical release. Further insertion of the forceps allows identification of the space between the A1 and A2 pulleys. This step is carefully monitored with ultrasound in both axial and sagittal views. While not mandatory, marking the A2 pulley's proximal edge, situated over the proximal phalanx, can be helpful. It is crucial to verify the forceps' position and orientation using ultrasound before proceeding with the surgical knife.

After precisely positioning the blunt mosquito forceps, a specialized surgical knife (Kemis ®H1, Newclip Technics®) is introduced. This knife features an extended "lower leg" designed to seamlessly in between the flexor tendon and flexor tendon sheath. The "upper leg" of this knife entraps the pulley. The mechanism of this cutting process, along with the knife's design is demonstrated in Fig. 4.5. Before commencing the release of the A1 pulley, it is imperative to verify the knife's exact central placement in both sagittal and axial views. Leveraging the knife toward the skin helps ensure the secure entrapment of the pulley. For optimal results, maintain the finger extended and maneuver the knife parallel to the flexor tendon while continuously monitoring the cutting process via ultrasound. This approach guarantees a safe, stable, and

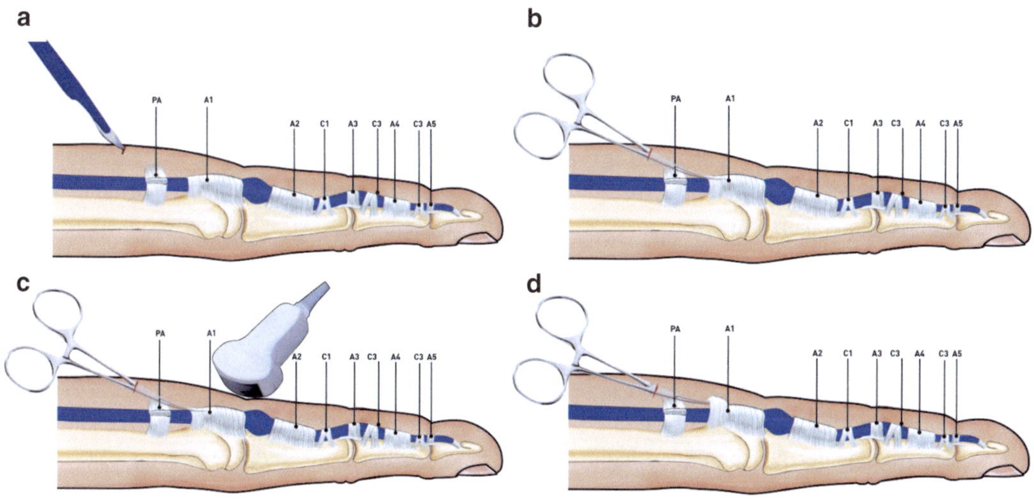

Fig. 4.4 (**a**) Small stab incision 0.5 cm proximal to the proximal edge of the pulley. (**b**) Blunt mosquito insertion into the flexor tendon sheath. (**c**) Verification of the direction and position of the mosquito with ultrasound. (**d**) Palpation of the pulley by pulling the mosquito upward

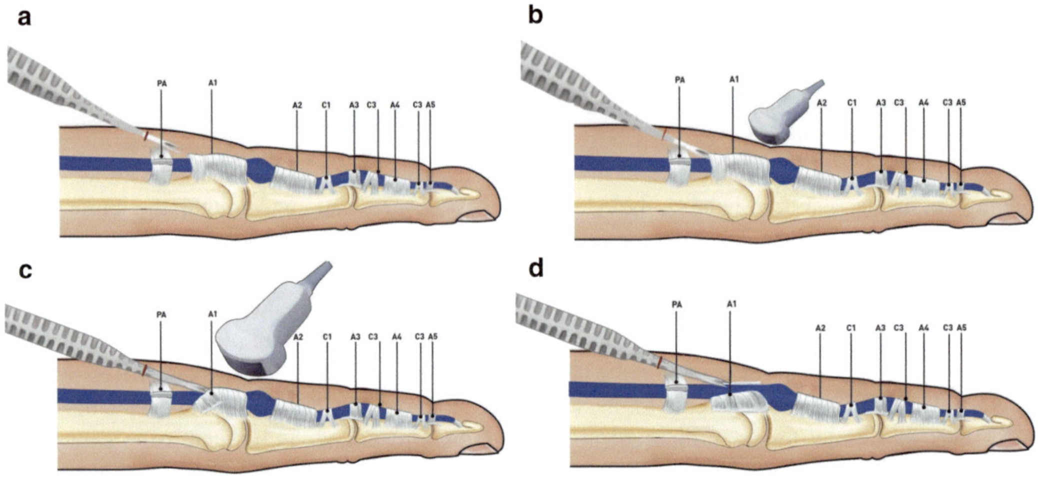

Fig. 4.5 Illustration and concept of the minimal invasive surgical knife (H1 kemis). After introduction of the knife (**a**), the longer leg of the knife is positioned underneath the A1 pulley (**b**). By sliding the knife deeper tangential to the flexor tendons and lifting it toward the skin, the pulley is entrapped in between the two legs of the knife (**c**). Cut tangential to the flexor tendons with the finger in extension and verify your position on ultrasound to obtain a full pulley release. A full release is felt as a drop of resistance (**d**)

thorough transection of the pulley. The successful release of the A1 pulley is indicated by a characteristic crisping sound and a modest resistance. A noticeable reduction in resistance signifies the completion of the pulley release. Ultrasound landmarks, such as the bony beak of the proximal phalanx (P1), are useful for confirming the A1 pulley's distal border (as shown in Fig. 4.3). The small stab incision should be left open rather than closed. This approach promotes healing within 3–5 days and enables spontaneous drainage of the initial hematoma, resulting in reduced pain and swelling.

4.7 Pearls and Pitfalls

To prevent incomplete trigger finger release at the A1 pulley, minimally invasive surgical knives are more effective than needle techniques that merely scratch the pulley fibers. Complete sectioning of the A1 pulley is ensured after the knife's passage. Ensuring the central position of the forceps and knife via ultrasound is key. Once positioned correctly, the knife entraps the pulley's proximal edge, marked by a crisping sound and slight resistance during release.

Post-release, complete sectioning of the A1 pulley is confirmed by the ease of moving reinserted forceps between the tendon and skin, verified by ultrasound, with a transverse view. In WALANT anesthesia cases, the patient's ability to flex and extend the finger without triggering confirms success. Additionally, observing the normal tenodesis cascade of the hand when moving the wrist from extension to flexion assures full release.

To avoid neurovascular damage, which was not observed in our series, several precautions are essential. Firstly, marking the flexor tendon direction on the skin, especially for the small finger, is critical. Secondly, verifying the central position of both forceps and knives with ultrasound guidance is vital (Fig. 4.6).

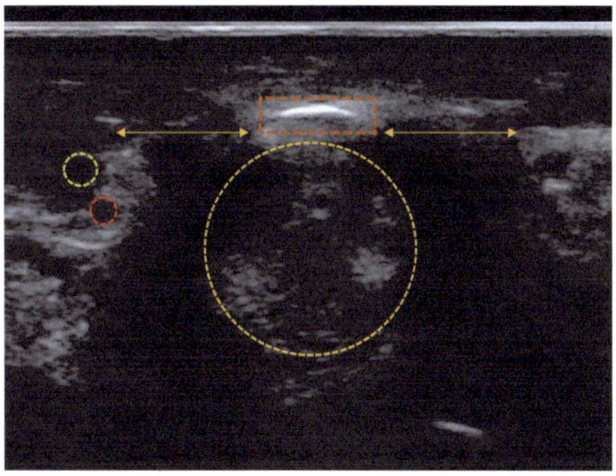

Fig. 4.6 Axial ultrasound view of the finger and flexor tendon (orange dotted line) with the surgical instrument in a central position between the flexor tendon and A1 pulley. Always ensure a central position of your instrument during the procedure by switching your probe to an axial out-of-plane view. The neurovascular structures (yellow and red dotted lines are a safe distance of your knife)

4.8 Postoperative Care and Outcomes

Postoperative care involves a small local bandage for 2–3 days, after which it can be removed. The percutaneous entry is left unsutured, and patients are encouraged to use their hands immediately for daily activities, emphasizing full finger extension and flexion. Patients typically experience rapid recovery with early return to daily activities.

In our recent series of 248 cases, we have not seen any persistent or recurrent triggering, and notably, we have observed no serious complications including infections, tendon injuries, or neurovascular damage. Scarring has not been a concern, contributing to patient satisfaction.

Approximately 8% of our patients, particularly those with significant preoperative synovitis or PIP joint contracture, may experience persistent local discomfort or motion limitations. However, these issues generally diminish by the 3-month mark—a point we communicate clearly to patients preoperatively to align their expectations. On rare occasions, a postoperative corticosteroid injection may be necessary, which typically leads to symptom resolution.

Take-Home Messages

Indication

Patient with surgery indications for long trigger finger.

After the failure of the medical treatment.

Contraindication:

Patients with strong deformity of the PIP joint, a risk of insufficient release.

Surgical Technique

(a) WALANT anesthesia 5/10CC; from the proximal flexion crease to the PIP joint.
(b) The measure of the length of P1 is done and reported from the flexion crease more proximally; it would represent the A1 pulley.
(c) Find the best entry point with a 25-gauge needle on the axis of the finger and the carpal tunnel. The entry point should be 5 mm proximal if the measure is done in B. The probe assesses the good position of the needle on a transverse view: to be far away from the neurovascular bundle; and on a plane view to be under the pulley.
(d) Open the skin with a knife to 1 cm.
(e) Pass a Halstead forceps under the skin to feel the A1 pulley. The probe assesses the good position of the forceps as in C.
(f) The mini knife is inserted with the long part that should be engaged under the pulley.
(g) In-plane and out-of-plane views are realized to ensure the goop position of the knife.
(h) The section is done on an in-plane view to control the full l release of the pulley.
(i) Control the release with a Halstead forceps.

Postoperative care

(a) Pressure dressing for 48 h

4.9 Conclusion

Ultrasound release of the long finger is feasible with this mini-invasive technique. The recovery is faster than open surgery. The main risk is an incomplete release.

Bibliography

1. Gil JA, Hresko AM, Weiss APC. Current concepts in the management of trigger finger in adults. J Am Acad Orthop Surg. 2020;28(15):e642–50.
2. Brozovich N, Agrawal D, Reddy G. A critical appraisal of adult trigger finger: pathophysiology, treatment, and future outlook. Plast Reconstr Surg Glob Open. 2019;7(8):e2360.
3. Fowler JR, Baratz ME. Percutaneous trigger finger release. J Hand Surg. 2013;38(10):2005–8.
4. Lorthioir JJR. Surgical treatment of trigger-finger by a subcutaneous method. JBJS. 1958;40(4)
5. Makkouk AH, Oetgen ME, Swigart CR, Dodds SD. Trigger finger: etiology, evaluation, and treatment. Curr Rev Musculoskelet Med. 2008;1(2):92–6.
6. Newport ML, Lane LB, Stuchin SA, York N. Treatment of trigger finger by steroid injection. J Hand Surg Am. 1990;15(5):748–50.
7. Grandizio LC, Speeckaert A, Brothers J, Graham J, Klena JC. Predictors of recurrence after corticosteroid injection for trigger digits. Hand (N Y). 2017;12(4):352.
8. Flensted F, Jensen CH, Daugaard H, Vedel JC, Jorgensen RW. Factors associated with increased risk of recurrence following treatment of trigger finger with corticosteroid injection. J Hand Microsurg. 2021;13(2):109–13.
9. Gilberts EC, Beekman WH, Stevens HJ, Wereldsma JC. Prospective randomized trial of open versus percutaneous surgery for trigger digits. J Hand Surg Am. 2001;26(3):497–500.
10. Wang J, Zhao JG, Liang CC. Percutaneous release, open surgery, or corticosteroid injection, which is the best treatment method for trigger digits? Clin Orthop Relat Res [Internet]. 2013;471(6):1879–86.
11. Le Viet D, Tsionos I, Boulouednine M, Hannouche D. Trigger finger treatment by ulnar superficialis slip resection (U.S.S.R.). J Hand Surg Br. 2004;29(4):368–73.
12. Fiorini HJ, Santos JBG, Hirakawa CK, Sato ES, Faloppa F, Albertoni WM. Anatomical study of the A1 pulley: length and location by means of cutaneous landmarks on the palmar surface. J Hand Surg Am [Internet]. 2011;36(3):464–8.
13. Jurbala B, Burbank T. Sonographic location of distal A1 pulley by means of a bony acoustic landmark on the proximal phalanx: an anatomic study. J Hand Surg Am. 2022;47(3):289.e1–6.

5 Retrograde Ultrasound-Guided Trigger Thumb Release

Francisco Javier Ferreira, Vincent Martinel, and Olivier Marès

5.1 Introduction

Trigger finger, also known as stenosing tenosynovitis, is characterized by the inability to smoothly flex or extend the affected digit, often resulting in a "triggering" sensation. This condition can affect any finger, but it is most commonly observed in the thumb and the ring finger. The thumb trigger finger refers explicitly to the manifestation of this condition in the thumb, where the flexor tendon becomes entrapped at the A1 pulley, leading to pain and restricted movement [1, 2].

The etiology of the trigger finger involves several factors, including repetitive use, inflammation, and anatomical variations that may lead to a thickened A1 pulley or tendon sheath. The thumb is more frequently affected due to its unique anatomical and functional characteristics, which include a greater range of motion and the significant role it plays in hand function.

Studies have shown that the incidence of trigger thumb is notably higher than that of trigger fingers in other digits, with some reports indicating that the thumb can be involved in up to 50% of cases of trigger finger [2, 3].

Clinically, the trigger thumb presents with symptoms such as pain at the base of the thumb, a palpable nodule, and a locking sensation during movement. Patients may experience difficulty in extending the thumb after it has been flexed, which can significantly impact daily activities and overall hand function.

5.2 Diagnosis

Diagnosis is typically made through clinical examination, and imaging studies such as ultrasound or MRI may be used to assess the condition of the tendon and pulley system [4].

Ultrasound imaging plays a pivotal role in diagnosing trigger finger by providing detailed visualization of the anatomical structures involved. Typical ultrasound findings include thickening of the A1 pulley, often observed as a nodular shape or global hypoechogenicity. Additionally, Doppler ultrasound may reveal hyperemia of the pulley, indicating increased blood flow associated with inflammation. In

Supplementary Information The online version contains supplementary material available at https://doi.org/10.1007/978-3-031-88679-9_5.

F. J. Ferreira (✉)
Hospital Universitario San Rafael, Madrid, Spain

International Chair of Musculoskeletal Ultrasound. UCAM, Murcia, Spain
e-mail: javierferreira@drjavierferreira.com

V. Martinel
Clinique de l'ormeau, Tarbes, France

O. Marès
Department of Traumatology and Orthopedic Surgery, University Hospital Nîmes, Nîmes, France

O. Marès et al. (eds.), *Ultrasound-Guided Limb Surgery*,
https://doi.org/10.1007/978-3-031-88679-9_5

advanced cases, cystic changes may be noted within the pulley, further complicating the condition [5, 6].

The dynamic assessment of the flexor tendon during finger motion can also highlight irregularities in tendon gliding, characteristic of trigger finger.

5.3 Treatment

The management of the trigger finger can be divided into conservative and surgical approaches. Conservative treatments typically include corticosteroid injections, splinting, and physiotherapy. Corticosteroid injections are often the first-line intervention due to their anti-inflammatory properties, which have been shown to effectively alleviate symptoms in many cases, with a reported success rate of up to 93% [7].

However, the efficacy of corticosteroid injections may decrease as the duration of symptoms exceeds 4 to 6 months. Also, the long-term effectiveness of repeated corticosteroid injections is debated, as a significant proportion of patients may require surgical intervention if symptoms persist [8].

When conservative treatments fail, surgical options become necessary.

5.3.1 Surgical Treatment

The most common surgical procedure for treating trigger finger is the open release of the A1 pulley, which has a remarkably high success rate of 97–99%. The effectiveness of this surgery relies on the clinician's precise anatomical knowledge and ability to anticipate the relevant surface landmarks. Gnanasekaran et al. [9] conducted an anatomical study to identify palmar surface landmarks that could guide the localization of the thumb's A1, A2, oblique, and variable annular pulleys. Their findings indicated that the proximal edge of the A1 pulley is situated 2 mm proximal to the proximal palmar crease. In comparison, the distal edge is positioned 3 mm distal to the proximal palmar crease. Additionally, the proximal variable annular and oblique pulleys were found to be 8 and 16 mm distal to the proximal palmar crease, respectively. The proximal edge of the A2 pulley was 3 mm proximal to the distal crease. Precise placement of the surgical incision over the A1 pulley of the thumb, combined with a careful surgical technique, is critical to avoid injury to the radial digital nerve, which may course obliquely beneath the incision and is considered the most vulnerable structure during this procedure.

The radial digital nerve is the structure most at risk during the open surgical release of the A1 pulley of the thumb. This is particularly true when a transverse incision is made at the level of the proximal palmar crease, as the radial collateral nerve lies near the incision site, situated only 1.29 mm deep to the skin surface and 0.67 mm anterior to the radial sesamoid bone.

Alternative surgical techniques, such as percutaneous release, have gained popularity. Ultrasound-guided thumb trigger finger release has emerged as a minimally invasive technique for trigger thumb release. This method has gained traction due to its safety, effectiveness, and reduced recovery time compared to traditional open surgical methods [10, 11].

5.3.2 Retrograde A1 Release Technique

Patients with a diagnosis of trigger thumb who have not responded to conservative treatment are eligible candidates for ultrasound-guided percutaneous release, analogous to those selected for open surgical intervention.

Patients with fused metacarpophalangeal or trapeziometacarpal joints may be contraindicated for the procedure, as the inability to extend these joints can complicate the release of the A1 pulley.

5.3.2.1 Prerequisites

Before the ultrasound-guided procedure, a comprehensive ultrasound assessment should be conducted using a linear, high-frequency transducer. Owing to the unique positioning of the thumb about the other fingers and the palm, a transducer with a small footprint is necessary.

This evaluation is critical for assessing pertinent structures, including the radial collateral nerve, which traverses the flexor pollicis longus tendon sheath obliquely, typically proximal to the A1 pulley.

5.3.2.2 Setup

Surgery is performed under wide awake local anesthesia with no tourniquet (WALANT). A 2 ml of 1% lidocaine with 1:100.000 epinephrine buffered with 1 ml of 8.4% sodium bicarbonate is injected under the skin at the PPC and another 2 ml at the DPC of the thumb.

The surgical field is prepared with two small sterile drapes, one with an opening. The surgeon wears sterile gloves. A 23 or 25G needle is used to visualize the ultrasound entry portal, and a 15-blade scalpel is utilized to create the portal. Stevens scissors with blunt atraumatic tips, mosquito forceps, and Adson forceps can be useful during the procedure to create the pathway. A needle holder is only required if skin closure with sutures is necessary.

The patient is positioned supine in the operating room, with the shoulder abducted 90 degrees, the elbow fully extended, and the forearm supinated and resting on an arm board. The thumb is slightly abducted, and an assistant extends the metacarpophalangeal and interphalangeal joints throughout the procedure.

The skin is cleaned with chlorhexidine.

The US probe is introduced in a sterile cover, and sterile gel or chlorhexidine is used between the skin and the probe to avoid air interference.

The landmarks for the surgical procedure are drawn on the skin with a sterile marker (Fig. 5.1). Hazani et al. [12] described the safest direction of longitudinal release of the pulley toward the hook of the hamate, which we must address under ultrasound.

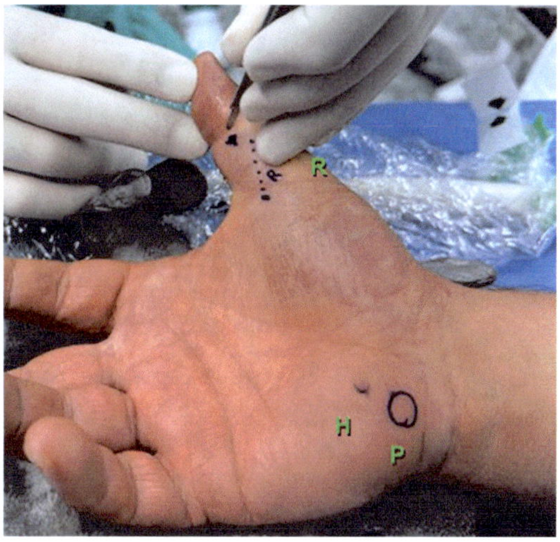

Fig. 5.1 Skin marks for ultrasound-guided trigger thumb release. R radial collateral nerve; P pisiform bone; H hamate hook tip

5.3.2.3 Surgery (Video 1)

A 25G needle is introduced under US guidance about 15 mm proximal to the PPC to avoid damage to the distal attachment of the oblique pulley and 2 mm radial from the center of the finger (Fig. 5.2). Once the proper location is checked under ultrasound, a small transverse incision of 1–2 mm is made. A blunt tip Stevens scissors are introduced inside the flexor pollicis longus (FPL) tendon sheath.

Next, the cutting device (Kemis H1®, NewClip Techniques®) is introduced into the ultrasound portal inside the FPL sheath, and the A1 annular pulley is retrogradely transected from distal to proximal toward the hook of the hamate under ultrasound short-axis and long-axis views, controlling the radial collateral nerve position.

Under ultrasound control, mosquito forceps inside the FPL sheath are used to check the complete release of the A1 pulley. Clinical triggering is also ruled out by asking the patient to flex and extend the thumb.

No stitches are used. The skin incision is closed with a 1/4-in. steri-strip, and a Bow-Tie-Type band-aid is applied.

The closure of the surgical wound is not performed, covering it with a small dressing.

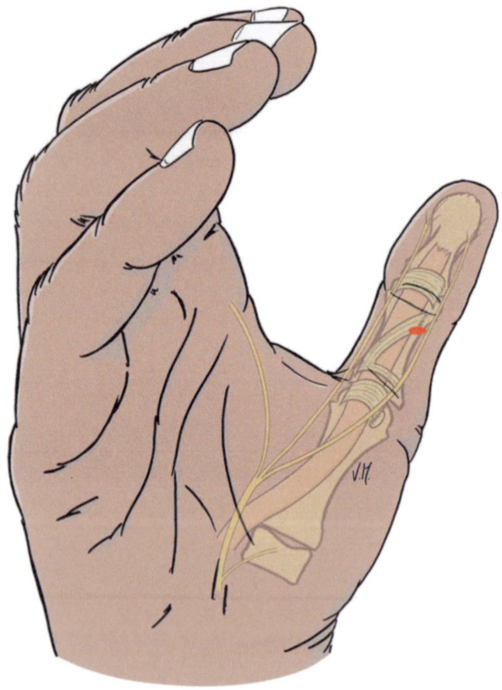

Fig. 5.2 Drawing showing the ultrasound entry portal at the thumb (red spot). Artwork by Vincent Martinel, reproduced with permission

5.3.2.4 Postoperative Care

Wound home care instructions are provided.

Patients are advised to perform tendon gliding exercises targeting the thumb and wrist. They may resume their usual daily activities without limitation but should refrain from excessive use during the initial 3-week recovery period.

Painkillers are prescribed for postoperative pain, especially the first 2 or 3 days.

Take-Home Messages

Indication

Thumb trigger finger

Contraindication: MP or TMC fusion

Surgical technique

Ultrasound-guided experienced surgeon with ultrasound-guided long trigger finger release

Identify skin and mark out surface landmarks.

Verify the hook of hamate location with ultrasound and mark on the skin.

Diagnostic ultrasound exam to confirm thickening of A1 pulley, locate and map the radial digital nerve, and confirm the location and trajectory of the tendon sheath.

Inject through a single portal raising a superficial wheel with 1.5 cc of local just proximal to the PP skin crease and use ultrasound guidance to directly inject 0.2 to 0.5 cc of local into the tendon sheath just proximal to A1 pulley.

Use a pair of Stevens Scissors to sound out the entry site into the tendon sheath.

Switch the scissors for the mosquito forceps to ensure you are inside the tendon sheath.

Advance the knife toward the hook of the hamate while simultaneously actuating it 30 to 60 degrees clockwise and counterclockwise to smoothly effect the release.

Check always the position of the radial collateral nerve of the thumb.

Use the mosquito forceps to verify the completeness of the release under direct ultrasound visualization in the short and long axis.

Postoperative care

Immediate fully light activity

Remove bandage at 24 hours PO

No need for any formal rehabilitation or physiotherapy.

Quick return to activities (2 weeks)

References

1. Moon W, Suh SW, Kim IC. Trigger digits in children. 2001;26(1):11–2. https://doi.org/10.1054/jhsb.2000.0417.
2. Chang EY, Chen KC, Chung CB. MR imaging findings of trigger thumb. 2015;44(8):1201–7. https://doi.org/10.1007/s00256-015-2172-y.
3. Shafaee-Khanghah Y, Akbari H, Bagheri N. Prevalence of carpal tunnel release as a risk factor of trigger finger. 2020;9(2):174–8. https://doi.org/10.29252/wjps.9.2.174.

4. Zhu W, et al. The cross-sectional area ratio of a specific part of the flexor pollicis longus tendon-a stable sonographic measurement for trigger thumb: a cross-sectional trial. 2023;24(1) https://doi.org/10.1186/s12891-023-06316-x.
5. Jia W, Zhao J, Liang C-C. Percutaneous release, open surgery, or corticosteroid injection, which is the best treatment method for trigger digits? 2013;471(6):1879–86. https://doi.org/10.1007/s11999-012-2716-6.
6. Wojahn RD, Foeger NC, Gelberman RH, Calfee RP. Long-term outcomes following a single corticosteroid injection for trigger finger. 2014;96(22):1849–54. https://doi.org/10.2106/jbjs.n.00004.
7. Dardas AZ, VandenBerg J, Shen T, Gelberman RH, Calfee RP. Long-term effectiveness of repeat corticosteroid injections for trigger finger. J Hand Surg. 2017;42(4):227–35. https://doi.org/10.1016/j.jhsa.2017.02.001.
8. Hollins AW, et al. Symptom duration and diabetic control influence success of steroid injection in trigger finger. Plast Reconstr Surg. 2022;150(2):357e–63e. https://doi.org/10.1097/prs.0000000000009320.
9. Gnanasekaran D, Veeramani R, Karuppusamy A. Topographic anatomical landmarks for pulley system of the thumb. Surg Radiol Anat. 2018;40(9):1007–12. https://doi.org/10.1007/s00276-018-2029-x.
10. Garcia HRP, Mund E, Romeiro P. Ultrasound-guided vs. non-guided trigger finger release: a systematic review and meta-analysis. Int Orthop. 2024;48(9):1–9. https://doi.org/10.1007/s00264-024-06243-z.
11. Nakagawa H, et al. Ultrasound-guided A1 pulley release: a systematic review. J Ultrasound Med. 2023;42(11):2491–9. https://doi.org/10.1002/jum.16294.
12. Hazani R, Whitney RD, Redstone J, Chowdhry S, Wilhelmi BJ. Safe treatment of trigger thumb with longitudinal anatomic landmarks. Eplasty. 2010;10

Dupuytren's Disease

6

Homid Fahandezh-Saddi Díaz,
Manuel Villanueva Martínez,
and Álvaro Iborra Marcos

6.1 Introduction

Palmar fibromatosis, also known as Dupuytren's disease or Dupuytren's contracture, is a benign fibroproliferative disorder in which subcutaneous fibrous nodules arise within the palmar fascia of the hand, eventually forming cordlike attachments with the adjacent flexor tendons [1–4].

Progressive shortening of these cordlike attachments ultimately results in flexion contractures of the fingers.

Palmar fibromatosis is common, affecting approximately 20% of people older than 65 years, and is associated with other fibromatoses, as well as diabetes mellitus types 1 and 2, alcoholism, and epilepsy. Although an underlying genetic predisposition and a higher prevalence in white Caucasic people are supported by twin and family studies, a multifactorial etiology is suggested by additional studies implicating trauma, microvascular injury, and immunologic processes [1–3].

Ultrasound (US) may be used to confirm palmar fibromatosis and for imaging-guided treatment [5–7]. Ultrasound guidance is used for collagenase injection therapy or surgical procedures to avoid complications of tendons and neurovascular structures [7].

6.2 Diagnosis

Palmar fibromatosis lesions most commonly affect the fourth digit, followed by the third, fifth, second, and first digits in decreasing order of frequency.

On US, the lesions are typically located superficial to the flexor tendons (93%) with their epicenter in the distal metacarpal zone (89%).

Dupuytren lesions are characteristically hypoechoic (98%) and noncompressible (95%) [5].

Sometimes, atypical features such as intralesional calcification (2%), compressibility (5%), and hyperemia on color Doppler imaging (6%) can be found.

Also, we can find lesions more distally than typical, at the metacarpophalangeal joint and proximal phalanx level. Less frequent lesions can

Supplementary Information The online version contains supplementary material available at https://doi.org/10.1007/978-3-031-88679-9_6.

H. F.-S. Díaz (✉) · M. V. Martínez
Orthopedic Surgery & Traumatology. Clínica AVANFI, Madrid, Spain

Á. I. Marcos
Podiatrist, Clínica AVANFI, Madrid, Spain

O. Marès et al. (eds.), *Ultrasound-Guided Limb Surgery*,
https://doi.org/10.1007/978-3-031-88679-9_6

be located superficial but lateral to the flexor tendons, rather than directly superficial to them [5].

Several benign and malignant lesions in the hand may simulate palmar fibromatosis: epithelioid sarcomas, giant cell tumors of the tendon sheath, ganglion cysts, inclusion cysts, stenosing tenosynovitis without triggering, edematous changes of the hand, and hyperkeratosis related to occupational activity [3]. Familiarity with the imaging features of palmar fibromatosis can aid in distinguishing it from these entities.

6.3 Treatment

During the past 10 years, complications and long-term postoperative recovery associated with limited fasciectomy (LF) have led to the use of minimally invasive techniques, including collagenase injections and percutaneous needle aponeurotomy (PNA) [5–12].

A systematic review of the literature demonstrates an overall complication rate below 4% with percutaneous needle aponeurotomy (PNA). The most common complication are skin tears, which may occur in 4% to 16% of cases, with tendon damage or complex regional pain syndrome being exceptional. Complication rate may be lower in non-advanced forms and when the surgeons are expert in the technique [8–17].

Because the cord must be palpable as a prerequisite before blind techniques are applied, most authors do not use ultrasound. Joint contracture is considered as a relative limitation for needle aponeurotomy, as it is the absence of a palpable cord [8–10, 17].

6.3.1 Personal Technique Surgical Procedure of Dupuytren's Disease

We have recently described our technique and results of ultrasound-guided aponeurotomy (USGA) and interphalangeal capsule release in patients with Dupuytren's disease [5, 6]. Ultrasound allows direct visualization of the cords and control of the flexor tendons and neurovascular bundle. Even in cases with interphalangeal joint contracture, we can release the capsule while preserving these structures.

6.3.1.1 Setup

The instrument set included a series of needles (22G, 21G, 18G, and 16G), a V-shaped straight curette, a blunt dissector, and an ultrasound device with a 10 to 17 MHz linear transducer. Hockey stick probe may be recommended for contractures over 80°, as normal linear probes may be difficult to adapt.

The patient is placed in the supine position with the hand resting on an arm board and facing upward. It is not necessary to apply a tourniquet. We do not use a malleable hand retractor, since we perform the procedure with two surgeons, as with other ultrasound-guided procedures we perform [5, 6].

6.3.1.2 Surgery (Video 1)

The cords are palpated and then identified with the probe in both the transverse plane and the longitudinal plane. We mark the cord pathway and select several entry points, from proximal to distal, between the metacarpal and the interphalangeal zone. Skin areas without severe retraction are preferred.

The portals are chosen on the ulnar side of the ray with the probe over the cord. (Fig. 6.1a–c).

The tendons, nerves, and vessels are always under direct control of the surgeons (Fig. 6.2a, b).

The needle and the syringe loaded with anesthetic (lidocaine 1% adrenaline 1/100,000) are used as a scalpel. First in the selected portal, we insert a little of anesthetic close to the cord.

With the probe in the transverse plane, we insert the needle under direct visualization from a (ulnar) entry point, rather than making multiple and blind perpendicular punctures as done in non-ultrasound-guided aponeurotomy. We make

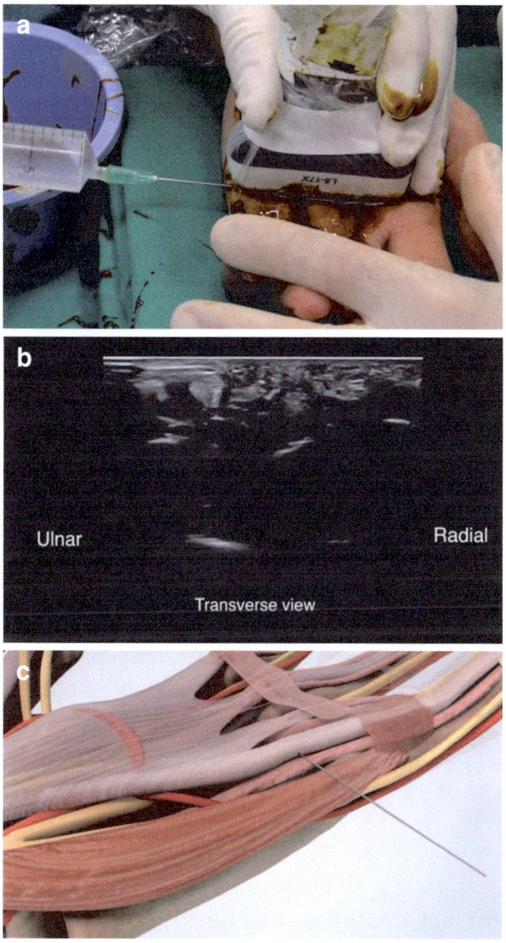

Fig. 6.1 (**a**) With the probe in the transverse plane, we insert the needle under direct visualization from an ulnar entry point. (**b**) The tendons, nerves, and vessels are always under direct control of the surgeons. The needles are used as a scalpel to do perforations to the cord. (**c**) 3D representation showing the procedure: the needle insert in the cord

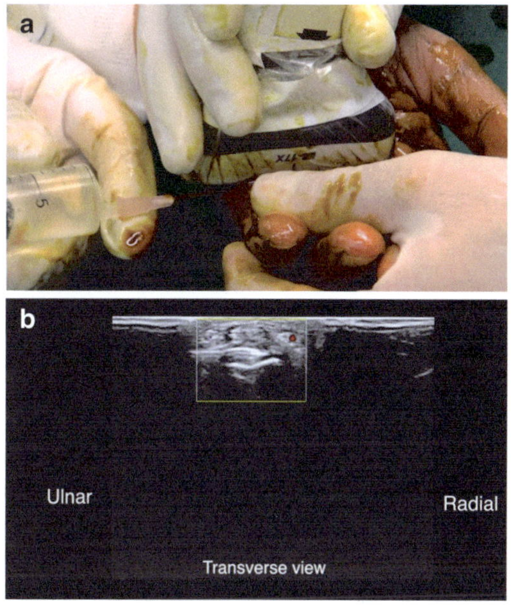

Fig. 6.2 (**a**) The tendons, nerves, and vessels are always under the direct control of the surgeons. Probe in the transverse plane. (**b**) The tendons, nerves, and vessels are always under the direct control of the surgeons with ultrasound. Probe in the transverse plane with Doppler mode to check the neurovascular bundle. We can see the needle under the flexor tendon and vessels

several portals starting proximal and moving distal, toward the fingers.

The movement of the needle is monitored at all times with US. The procedure can be performed with different thicknesses needles. The needle is inserted from ulnar to radial at the point selected, with the transducer placed "in-plane" with the needle along the short axis of the cord. Multiple perforations are made from ulnar to radial and from deep to superficial at all selected points until the cord is released.

Reducing the tension of the cords at several points minimizes skin complications when the fingers are extended. The depth of the needle and its position with respect to vessels and nerves can be controlled using ultrasound B mode and Doppler mode in "in-plane" and "out-of-plane" view.

Skin retractions into the subcutaneous tissue are released by severing the diseased fibers that insert into the dermis by moving the needle or the curette following a horizontal windshield wiper motion in the plane just below the skin.

After a first phase of multiple horizontal perforations from ulnar to radial, we start making a levering movement from deep to superficial, and the sharp bevel of this needle cuts the cord like a knife. It is very important to maintain the position of the needle and the probe with the cord under tension in the same plane while making the perforations, because if the tension is released, the original plane of the needle will be lost, rendering the aponeurotomy more difficult [1].

Interphalangeal contracture is a problematic issue with blind surgery. Ultrasound-guided surgery enables the contracture to be released with direct control of the nerves and vessels, by staying immediately beneath them. For this surgical gesture, we prefer 22G and 18G needles [5, 17].

When we feel that the cord is sufficiently loose at several points or if we can pass the needle through it, we extend the finger and break the cord. The surgeon can feel the release of the cord like a snap. We complete the proximal cuts by flexing the fingers and extending the metacarpophalangeal joint, thus reducing skin tension. We complete the distal cuts by flexing the wrist and metacarpophalangeal joint and extending the finger [5, 6].

We can then check the final result and ask the patient to flex and extend his/her hand.

We can do bilateral cases with this technique at the same time [5, 6]. We can do this technique in the OR and recently we started to do it in the office. It is a reliable and safe technique.

We have treated almost 150 patients with excellent results, and we have already reported our results with the first 70 patients [5] (Figs. 6.3a, b and 6.4a, b).

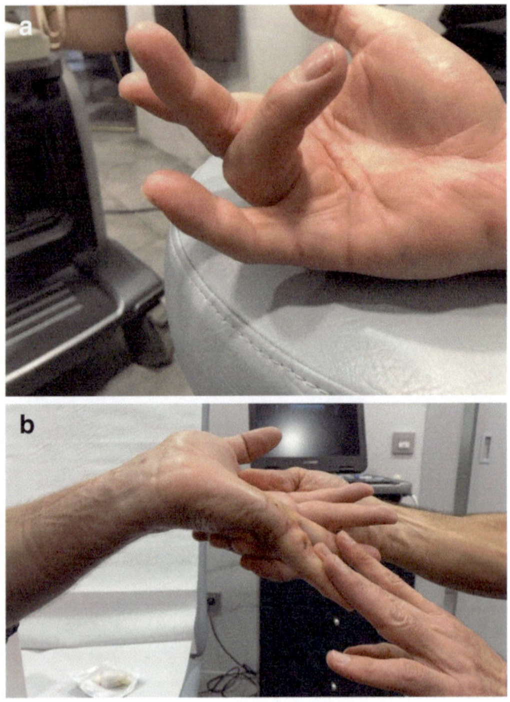

Fig. 6.3 (**a**) Dupuytren stage III of Tubiana affecting fourth and fifth fingers before the procedure. (**b**) Image after the ultrasound-guided aponeurotomy of the same digits

6.3.1.3 Postoperative Care

The patient can move the hand immediately after the procedure. No sutures are required. We use adhesive strips and an elastic bandage.

At 24–48 h, we remove the elastic bandage. In severe PIP contractures, hand therapist makes a splint and shows physiotherapy exercises.

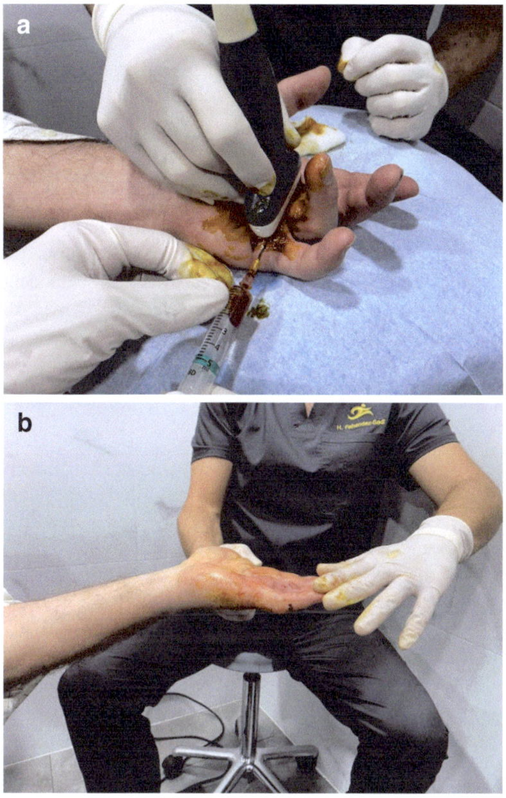

Fig. 6.4 (**a**) Dupuytren stage III of Tubiana affecting fourth finger before the procedure. (**b**) Image after the ultrasound-guided aponeurotomy of the same digits

6.4 Results

In our series recently publicated [5], the contractures were Tubiana stage I in 15 cases, stage II in 41, and stage III in 14 cases. In 21% of cases, the digits had isolated metacarpophalangeal joint contractures. Two cases (3%) involved an isolated proximal interphalangeal joint contracture (stage II). The remainder (53 fingers, 76%) involved contractures of both the metacarpophalangeal and proximal interphalangeal joints.

Proximal interphalangeal capsule release was performed in 15 cases with digital deformity (11 cases with Tubiana stage III and 4 patients with Tubiana stage II). Preoperative mean contracture was 70° (35–115°). Preoperative metacarpophalangeal joint contracture means 39° (range, 25–65°), and proximal interphalangeal contracture means 40° (range, 15–70°) (excluding the 15 cases with isolated metacarpophalangeal deformity).

The improvement after surgery means 67°, which represents 95% of the contracture.

Residual contractures mean 4° (0–15°). Metacarpophalangeal joint contractures were corrected with a mean of 37° (95% of the contracture) and proximal interphalangeal joint contractures with a mean of 38° (94.5% of the contracture) immediately after surgery (excluding the 15 cases with isolated metacarpophalangeal deformity).

At 1 and 2 years of follow-up, total correction mean 63°, which represents 90% of the initial global contracture. Correction for metacarpophalangeal joint contracture mean 35.3° (91.4%), and correction for proximal interphalangeal joint contracture (excluding the cases with isolated MCP deformity) mean 35°, which represents a correction of 88% of the initial contracture.

All patients were satisfied at 3 months of follow-up and 1 and 2 years of follow-up, with a rate of 9 on the visual analogue scale (0–10).

Take-Home Messages

Indication

Patients with Dupuytren's disease, Tubiana's stages I and II.

Stage III only for experienced surgeons

Contraindication

Patients with Dupuytren's disease, Tubiana's stage IV

Surgical Technique

US examination with a "hockey stick" probe and skin marking of the cord's pathway

Needle fasciotomy is performed from the ulnar side of the cord.

16G needle is used for cord fasciotomy and 18–22G needle is used for PIP release

Perform multiple cuts over the cord

Keep always the cord under tension until the fasiotomy is completed.

Postoperative care

Inmediate postop movement. No stitches are required

Splinting if severe PIP contractures are treated.

References

1. Lanting R, Broekstra DC, Werker PM, et al. A systematic review and meta-analysis on the prevalence of Dupuytren disease in the general population of Western countries. Plast Reconstr Surg. 2014;133(3):593–603.
2. Geoghegan JM, Forbes J, Clark DI, et al. Dupuytren's disease risk factors. J Hand Surg Br. 2004; 29(5):423–6
3. Shih B, Bayat A. Scientific understanding and clinical management of Dupuytren disease. Nat Rev Rheumatol. 2010;6:715–26.
4. Créteur V, Madani A, Gosset N. Ultrasound imaging of Dupuytren's contracture. J Radiol. 2010;91(6):687–91. https://doi.org/10.1016/s0221-0363(10)70098-6. PMID: 20808269.
5. Villanueva M, Iborra A, Fahandezh H, Sanz P, Noriega. Ultrasound-guided aponeurotomy and interphalangeal capsule release for treatment of Dupuytren's disease: A novel surgical approach. J Hand Surg. 2022 (European Volume):1–8
6. Villanueva M, Fahandezh H, Iborra A. Ultrasonographic-guided aponeurotomy for Dupuytren contracture. Orlando: AAOS Video Technique; 2022.
7. Chen NC, Srinivasan RC, Shauver MJ, et al. A systematic review of outcomes of fasciotomy, aponeurectomy, and collagenase treatments for Dupuytren's contracture. Hand. 2011;6:250–5.
8. Beaudreuil J, Lermusiaux JL, Teyssedou JP. Multineedle aponeurotomy for advanced Dupuytren's disease: a 16-month follow-up study (MNA 2 Study). J Hand Surg. 2012;37:795–6.
9. Hovius SE, Kan HJ, Verhoekx JS, Khouri RK. Percutaneous Aponeurotomy and Lipofilling (PALF): a regenerative approach to Dupuytren contracture. Clin Plast Surg. 2015;42(3):375–81.
10. Morhart M. Pearls and pitfalls of needle aponeurotomy in Dupuytren's disease. Plast Reconstr Surg. 2015;135(3):817–25.
11. Diaz R, Curtin C. Needle aponeurotomy for the treatment of Dupuytren's disease. Hand Clin. 2014;30(1):33–8.
12. Gerber RA, Perry R, Thompson R, et al. Dupuytren's contracture: a retrospective database analysis to assess clinical management and costs in England. BMC Musculoskelet Disord. 2011;12:73.
13. Zhou C, Selles RW, Slijper HP, Feitz R, van Kooij Y, Moojen TM, Hovius SE. Comparative effectiveness of percutaneous needle aponeurotomy and limited fasciectomy for Dupuytren's contracture: a multicenter observational study. Plast Reconstr Surg. 2016 Oct;138(4):837–46.
14. Van Rijssen AL, Gerbrandy FS, Ter Linden H, et al. A comparison of the direct outcomes of percutaneous needle fasciotomy and limited fasciectomy for Dupuytren's disease: a 6-week follow-up study. J Hand Surg Am. 2006;31:717–25.
15. Van Rijssen AL, ter Linden H, Werker PM. Five-year results of a randomized clinical trial on treatment in Dupuytren's disease: percutaneous fasciotomy versus limited fasciectomy. Plast Reconstr Surg. 2012;129:469–77.
16. Pess GM, Pess RM, Pess RA. Results of needle aponeurotomy for Dupuytren contracture in over 1,000 fingers. J Hand Surg Am. 2012;37:651–6.
17. Misra A, Jain A, Ghazanfar R, et al. Predicting the outcome of surgery for the proximal interphalangeal joint in Dupuytren's disease. J Hand Surg [Am]. 2007;32(2):240–5.

Part III

Wrist

7 Carpal Tunnel Injection and Hydrodissection

Francisco Javier Ferreira

7.1 Introduction

Carpal tunnel syndrome (CTS) does not refer to a disease, but to a constellation of symptoms that are produced by the compression of the median nerve as it passes through the carpal tunnel. It is one of the most common peripheral nerve disorders, with a population prevalence of 5.8% in women and 0.6% in men [1]. Although CTS has been considered a trivial condition, it causes a significant health problem. CTS and hearing impairment accounts for more morbidity, measured by cases and working days lost, than any other condition in the United States of America working population.

CTS continues to be an idiopathic syndrome, although there are several risk factors associated with this pathology. Environmental factors, such as obesity, work activity, alcohol and/or coffee consumption, tobacco, etc., are likely to have the greatest influence on the development of CTS. [2–4]

7.2 Physiopathology

CTS occurs as a result of a combination of the following events: increased pressure, tissue ischemia, and mechanical phenomena, which alter the normal physiology of the nerve within the carpal tunnel [5].

Edema of the median nerve is one of the main findings in CTS.

Chronic compression causes fibrosis and prevents slippage, damaging the mesoneurium, which results in adhesion of the nerve to the surrounding tissue, causing traction neuritis.

Alterations in the synovial tissue and subsynovial connective tissue (SSCT) lining the flexor tendons in the carpal tunnel are predisposing factors in the development of idiopathic CTS [6]. Synovial thickening and fibrosis of the subsynovial connective tissue are the most common histological changes in CTS and can be caused by repetitive maneuvers of the hand, increasing the tunnel pressure [7, 8].

Supplementary Information The online version contains supplementary material available at https://doi.org/10.1007/978-3-031-88679-9_7.

F. J. Ferreira (✉)
Hospital Universitario San Rafael, Madrid, Spain

International Chair of Musculoskeletal Ultrasound. UCAM, Murcia, Spain
e-mail: javierferreira@drjavierferreira.com

O. Marès et al. (eds.), *Ultrasound-Guided Limb Surgery*,
https://doi.org/10.1007/978-3-031-88679-9_7

7.3 Diagnosis

The mainstay of the diagnosis of CTS continues to be the patient's medical history, with night paresthesias as the most characteristic symptom.

Up to 66% of patients with CTS have sensitive imparment [9]. Weakness of the abductor pollicis brevis is the most sensitive motor sign, as it is rarely innervated by the ulnar nerve.

Specific tests, like Phalen and Durkan test, aim to reproduce or cease certain symptoms that patients with CTS typically suffer intermittently.

Most studies on the diagnosis of CTS accept nerve conduction studies as the gold standard [10].

Ultrasound is a useful tool in the diagnosis of CTS. As in any compressive neuropathy, an increase in nerve caliber and a decrease in echogenicity is observed, with the loss of the fascicular characteristic pattern, both at the point of compression and proximal to it. Ultrasound measurements of the median nerve cross-sectional area (CSA) at the carpal tunnel inlet are highly predictive of CTS, with optimal cutoff values identified for diagnosis, suggesting that ultrasound is comparable to electrophysiology in diagnosing CTS. [11]

Ultrasound elastography has been beneficial in diagnosing CTS, detecting changes in the median nerve that correlate with the condition. [12]

7.4 Conservative Treatment

Although CTS is generally considered to be a highly treatable condition, there is still scant evidence in relation to most of the existing treatments for CTS.

Patients using night splints usually experience improvement in symptoms after 2 weeks of use. [13]

The use of corticosteroid injections for the treatment of CTS is controversial. The mechanism of action of depot corticosteroids includes a decrease in the inflammatory reaction as they limit capillary dilation and vascular permeability. They also reduce the accumulation of polymorphonuclear leukocytes and macrophages, as well as the release of vasoactive enzymes [14].

Ultrasound-guided punctures achieve a better response, with a faster improvement in symptoms compared to conventional injections [15]. They also reduce post-puncture and infiltration pain, increasing the duration of the infiltration effect by more than 70%.

The definitive procedure of surgical decompression remains controversial, with an overall success rate of about 75% [16].The nonsurgical management has not been deeply studied, and several widely used treatments, for example, nonsteroidal anti-inflammatory agents, are supported by no class 1 trial evidence at all.

Steroids relieve local ischemia and reduce synovial swelling or vascular congestion in the carpal tunnel.

Nerve hydrodissection is a relatively new and promising ultrasound-guided technique that relies on hydrostatic forces from fluid injection adjacent to affected nerves to dissect them from the surrounding structures [17] and has been used for treatment of neuropathic pain [18].

Hydrodissection also reduce gliding resistance of the median nerve within the carpal tunnel, potentially benefiting patients with CTS [19].

The procedure can be performed through in-plane or out-of-plane approaches.

7.5 Personal Technique (Video 1)

7.5.1 Indications

Candidates for ultrasound-guided percutaneous release would be those diagnosed with CTS, without response to conventional conservative treatment with oral steroids and/or night splinting.

7.5.2 Prerequisites

A previous ultrasound study should be carried out with a linear, high-frequency probe (8.0–13.0 MHz desirable) for assessing anatomy of the carpal tunnel and address possible vascular or median nerve variants.

7.5.3 Procedure

The interventional procedure is performed at the office. Hydrodissection of the carpal tunnel is carried out with a high-frequency transducer (8.0–13.0 MHz).

Eleven cc of fluid is introduced inside the carpal tunnel. Fluid composition is 9 cc of saline, 1 cc of anesthetic (2% lidocaine), and 1 cc of triamcinolone acetate 40 mg (Trigon depot®). This composition is similar to that proposed by Malone et al. [20] Triamcinolone is used because it has shown significant alleviation of sensory disturbance, edema, inflammation, and pain-related peptide upregulation on entrapment neuropathy [21]. The technique is carried out utilizing two punctures with a 21G needle, following an aseptic technique, keeping the probe sterile by covering it with a transparent plastic adhesive dressing (Tegaderm®; 3 M® Health Care, USA), using Betadine gel® as a transducer gel. The examiner is also protected with sterile gloves. To reduce the discomfort of punctures, topical anesthesia of the puncture area is performed.

Both punctures are performed following an "in-plane" approach in order to be able to identify the needle along its entire path, especially at the level of the tip, preventing damage to neurovascular and tendon structures. The first puncture is performed using an ulnar approach to the wrist described by Smith et al. [22], to free the space between the median nerve and the flexor tendon compartment at the carpal tunnel inlet (Fig. 7.1).

Subsequently, another puncture is performed in a proximal to distal fashion, visualizing the nerve in its longitudinal or sagittal axis, to free the nerve from the retinacular ligament (Fig. 7.2).

Finally, disinfection of the puncture areas is carried out, covering it with adhesive dressings. No wrist immobilization is performed, although

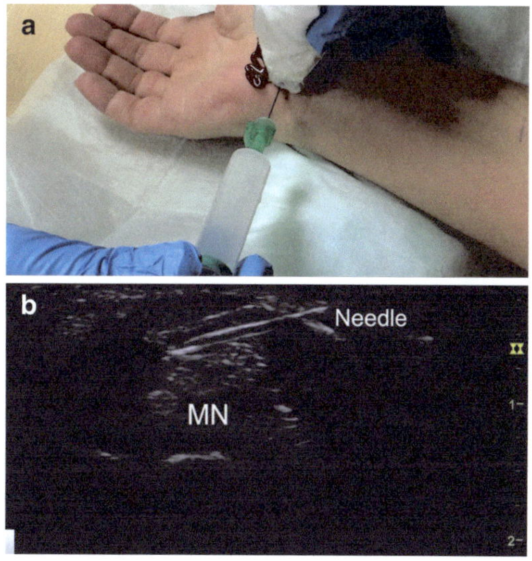

Fig. 7.1 (**a**) Clinical image of the ulnar approach of the carpal tunnel injection. (**b**) Ultrasound short-axis "in-plane" view

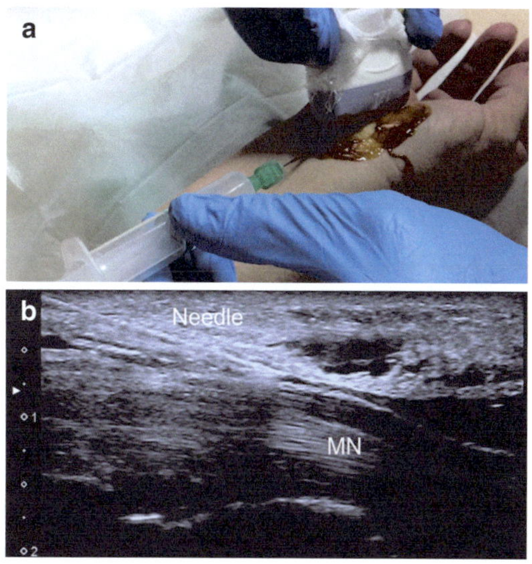

Fig. 7.2 (**a**) Clinical image of a proximal to distal injection of the carpal tunnel. (**b**) Ultrasound long-axis "in-plane" view

a 48-h relative rest is advice to minimize post-injection flare.

7.6 Results

We presented in 2019 at the XXIV Congress of the Spanish Society of Hand Surgery (SECMA) our results with 140 cases, with an average age of 55 years, 75% of whom were women. In the study, 24 cases were lost. Sixty-seven percent of the cases were diagnosed clinically and electromyographically as severe. Eighty-one percent were high demanding workers at a minimum of 1 year follow-up, and 58.8% had shown evident and stable improvement. Seventy percent of patients reported that they would do it again.

Although there are well-known side effects of local corticosteroid injections like tendon rupture, skin hypopigmentation, and fat atrophy, post-injection flare, and face flushing, we only recorded two patients with post-injection flare, and seven patients communicated face flushing.

Take-Home Messages

Indication:

Carpal tunnel syndrome

Contraindication

Active infection

Allergy to hydrodissection fluid components

Polyneuropathy

Technique:

(a) High-frequency linear probe. Office-based procedure
(b) Hydrodissection fluid: 9 cc of saline, 1 cc of anesthetic (2% lidocaine), and 1 cc of triamcinolone acetate 40 mg
(c) "In-plane" view. Ulnar approach and direct proximal and distal approach

Post-procedure care:

(a) Adhesive dressing
(b) Partial rest 24 h

References

1. de Krom MC, et al. Carpal tunnel syndrome: prevalence in the general population. J Clin Epidemiol. 1992;45:373–6.
2. Chell J, Stevens A, Davis TR. Work practices and histopathological changes in the tenosynovium and flexor retinaculum in carpal tunnel syndrome in women. J Bone Joint Surg Br. 1999;81:868–70.
3. Martin S. Carpal tunnel syndrome: a job-related risk. Am Pharm. 1991;Ns31:21–4.
4. Nathan PA, Meadows KD, Doyle LS. Occupation as a risk factor for impaired sensory conduction of the median nerve at the carpal tunnel. J Hand Surg. 1988;13:167–70.
5. Werner RA, Andary M. Carpal tunnel syndrome: pathophysiology and clinical neurophysiology. Clin Neurophysiol. 2002;113:1373–81.
6. Ettema AM, Zhao C, Amadio PC, O'Byrne MM, An KN. Gliding characteristics of flexor tendon and tenosynovium in carpal tunnel syndrome: a pilot study. Clin Anat. 2007;20:292–9.
7. Millesi H, Zöch G, Rath T. The gliding apparatus of peripheral nerve and its clinical significance. Ann De Chir De La Main Et Du Membre Supérieur. 1990;9:87–97.
8. Mackinnon SE. Pathophysiology of nerve compression. Hand Clin. 2002;18:231–41.
9. Spindler HA, Dellon AL. Nerve conduction studies and sensibility testing in carpal tunnel syndrome. J Hand Surg Am. 1982;7:260–3.
10. Jarvik JG, Yuen E. Diagnosis of carpal tunnel syndrome: electrodiagnostic and magnetic resonance imaging evaluation. Neurosurg Clin N Am. 2001;12:241–53.
11. Cartwright MS, et al. Evidence-based guideline: neuromuscular ultrasound for the diagnosis of carpal tunnel syndrome. Muscle Nerve. 2012;46:287–93.
12. Orman G, Ozben S, Huseyinoglu N, Duymus M, Orman KG. Ultrasound elastographic evaluation in the diagnosis of carpal tunnel syndrome: initial findings. Ultrasound Med Biol. 2013;39:1184–9.
13. Burke DT, Burke MM, Stewart GW, Cambre A. Splinting for carpal tunnel syndrome: in search of the optimal angle. Arch Phys Med Rehabil. 1994;75:1241–4.
14. Cole BJ, Schumacher RH Jr. Injectable corticosteroids in modern practice. J Am Acad Orthop Surg. 2005;13:37–46.
15. Ustun N, et al. Ultrasound-guided vs. blind steroid injections in carpal tunnel syndrome: a single-blind randomized prospective study. Am J Phys Med Rehabil. 2013;92:999–1004.
16. Bland JD. Treatment of carpal tunnel syndrome. Muscle Nerve. 2007;36:167–71.
17. Ferreira FJ, Pino JGD. Ultrasound-guided hydrodissection for severe carpal tunnel treatment. Hand. 2016;11:90S.
18. Lam SKH, Reeves KD, Cheng A-L. Transition from deep regional blocks toward deep nerve hydrodissec-

tion in the upper body and torso: method description and results from a retrospective chart review of the analgesic effect of 5% dextrose water as the primary hydrodissection injectate to enhance safety. Biomed Res Int. 2017;2017:7920438.
19. Evers S, et al. Corticosteroid injections for carpal tunnel syndrome: long-term follow-up in a population-based cohort. Plast Reconstr Surg. 2017;140:338–47.
20. Malone DG, Clark TB, Wei N. Ultrasound-guided percutaneous injection, hydrodissection, and fenestration for carpal tunnel syndrome: description of a new technique. J Appl Res. 2010;10:8.
21. Shibayama M, et al. The effects of locally injected triamcinolone on entrapment neuropathy in a rat chronic constriction injury model. J Hand Surg Am. 2014;39:1714–21.
22. Smith J, Wisniewski SJ, Finnoff JT, Payne JM. Sonographically guided carpal tunnel injections: the ulnar approach. J Ultrasound Med. 2008;27:1485–90.

8 Ultrasound-Guided Carpal Tunnel Release: Anterograde Technique

Olivier Marès, Lara Moscato,
and Pascal Kouyoumdjian

8.1 Introduction

Carpal tunnel syndrome is the most common mononeuropathy of the upper limb [1].

It results from compression of the median nerve as it passes through the carpal tunnel at the wrist. The carpal tunnel is an anatomical narrowing bounded at the front by the flexor retinaculum and at the rear by the carpal bones. In addition to the median nerve, this inextensible cavity contains the nine superficial and deep flexor tendons of the fingers. Following hormonal changes (menopause, diabetes, pregnancy) or repeated trauma, inflammatory synovitis can develop on the flexor tendons, leading to an increase in the volume of the carpal tunnel's contents and consequent compression of the median nerve [2]. Symptoms appear progressively. Sensory symptoms such as paresthesias in the median cutaneous sensory area are predominant, first nocturnal or positional, and then diurnal and finally constant. Sometimes they are accompanied with pain, which is often irradiated to the forearm. Some patients can develop a fix sensory loss. Thenar weakness and atrophy can appear specially in elderly patients. [1, 2]

8.2 Diagnosis

Diagnosis is based on both clinical examination and questioning of the patient. A history of diabetes, metabolic diseases, pregnancy, menopause, connective tissue diseases such as rheumatoid arthritis, etc. should be sought. Occupation, sports, and leisure activities should be recorded in the patient's file, in order to identify any repetitive or micro-traumatic gestures that may contribute to the condition [1, 2].

Tinel and Phalen provocation tests can be used to identify nocturnal symptoms in early-stage cases. A tripod force measurement can also be used to identify motor impairment. Scratch collapse test can also be useful.

Electromyography remains the gold standard for quantifying median nerve damage [3]. In severe cases, it helps to anticipate the potential for recovery, particularly in cases of advanced motor damage with muscular denervation and amyotrophy. A conduction velocity of less than 40 m/s on the sensory side at the exit of the carpal

Supplementary Information The online version contains supplementary material available at https://doi.org/10.1007/978-3-031-88679-9_8.

O. Marès (✉) · P. Kouyoumdjian
Department of Traumatology and Orthopedic Surgery, University Hospital Nîmes, Nîmes, France

L. Moscato
University Hospital Montpellier, Montpellier, France

O. Marès et al. (eds.), *Ultrasound-Guided Limb Surgery*,
https://doi.org/10.1007/978-3-031-88679-9_8

tunnel confirms the diagnosis of nerve compression. It can also unmask multistage compression, at the cervical spine or a polyneuropathy.

Ultrasound enables us to measure the volume of the median nerve, which may be increased upstream of the compression. A surface area greater than 12 mm^2 is considered to be indicative of nerve damage, with sensitivity and specificity similar to those of EMG [5].

Moreover ultrasound, especially when performed by the surgeon during the consultation, provides excellent visualization of the carpal tunnel's contents. Among other things, it enables us to identify potential anatomical variations in the median nerve [4] (bifid nerve, sub- or intra-ligamentary thenar branch, persistence of median nerve artery) and the palmar arch, so that we can propose appropriate and safe surgical management if indicated). We also look for rare causes of compression, such as synovial cysts or supernumerary muscles and tendons, which may require a different surgical approach [5].

8.3 Treatment

In the case of minor to moderate compression, medical treatment is the first choice. A nocturnal postural splint, a course of NSAIDs or oral corticoids, and relative rest of the wrist are the first measures to be implemented [1, 2]. Ultrasound-guided infiltration of cortisone derivatives can provide effective, long-lasting management if there are no contra-indications, but should not be repeated too often, due to its toxicity on tendon structures [1, 2].

8.4 Surgical Management

In the event of failure of medical treatment or severe compression, surgical release should be considered.

There are several surgical techniques, but all involve cutting the entire length of the annular carpal ligament to increase the volume of the carpal tunnel [6]. The ultrasound-guided technique [7] has developed considerably in recent years. Studies comparing these techniques have found no significant difference in postoperative functional results [8]. There are clearly identified risks, such as notable infection, incomplete release, and vascular or nerve lesions, but the complication rate does not appear to vary according to the technique used, when performed by an experienced surgeon. On the other hand, the learning curve is clearly greater for endoscopic and ultrasound techniques than for the open technique [8].

Today's patients are keen to undergo endoscopic surgery because of its ultra-minimally invasive nature, but this practice is costly in terms of equipment and resources [9]. Thanks to ultrasound, and the use of the WALANT anesthesia, we can now offer patients ultra-minimally invasive treatment in a simplified, safe surgery [10]. However, transposing US carpal tunnel release management to the office setting should only be done once we have acquired solid experience of ultrasound-guided procedure in the operating room and with selected patients so as not to unnecessarily increase the risk of complications [10].

8.5 Personal Technique

8.5.1 Prerequisites

During the diagnostic clinics, the surgeon performs an ultrasound evaluation to pinpoint the location of the nerve and eliminate any variations that might contraindicate ultrasound-guided liberation. The patient is reconvened to the office surgery in a dedicated slot. There is no need to fast or stop anticoagulant treatment. There is no need for a pre-anesthetic consultation.

8.5.2 Setup

Surgery is performed in an outpatient department under WALANT anesthesia. A mix of 10 ml of physiological serum and 10 ml of lidocaine with 1/100 epinephrine is prepared to obtain a 20 ml syringe. Anesthesia is administered from proximal to distal, with a single puncture point at the wrist's proximal flexion crease, gradually extending subcutaneously along the entire length of the annular ligament [11]. A further intra-canal injection is made with 5 mL of solution. The drape is limited to a "perforated field," with disinfection using biseptine.

The surgeon wears only a mask and sterile gloves and sets up his ultrasound equipment using a cover and single-use sterile gel.

8.5.3 Surgery (Video 1)

The wrist is positioned in slight extension by a band placed on the dorsal surface to facilitate focusing. Ultrasound tracking is performed along two axes using a high-frequency linear probe (12–18 mHz). The thenar motor branch must be localized to prevent any section. It is most often located extra-ligamentarily (75.2%) but may also be located sub-ligamentarily (13.5%) or trans-ligamentarily (11.3%).

A 5 mm transverse incision is made at the proximal flexion crease of the wrist, in line with the axis of the radial edge of the fourth finger. Under ultrasound control, the entire length of the annular ligament is dissected above and below, using Halstead forceps to limit the risk of tissue interposition and to detach the flexor synovium from the retinaculum. Next, a kemis knife® (NewClip Techincs®) is introduced under ultrasound control, for anterograde sectioning.

A transverse view is done to assure the good position of the kemis knife around the ligament to avoid any soft tissue to be in the knife. After, in a long-axis ultrasound view, the annular ligament is positioned between the two jaws of the knife to control the full section of the ligament. In a fluid, restrained movement, the retinaculum is sectioned along its entire length. The gesture is done under fully control of an in plane view where we tracked all the different anatomical structures such as the nerve branches and the palmar arch (by using the Doppler). Finally, a Halstead forceps is introduced under US control to check that the section has been performed completely. A simple dressing is applied with no use of any stiches or glue.

8.5.4 Postoperative Care

The dressing is removed 24 h after surgery, and no nursing care is required afterward.

No postoperative immobilization is required.
Driving and daily activities are immediately authorized.
No rehabilitation is prescribed.
The patient is given a 15-day sick leave and a prescription for Level 1 painkillers.

8.6 Conclusion

The simplification of the office surgery care pathway was made possible by performing the procedure under WALANT anesthesia and with an ultrasound-guided technique. According to the results of studies carried out in our unit, this pathway led to increased patient satisfaction compared with care in the operating room [12]. We were also able to demonstrate a reduction in costs compared with Agee endoscopic surgery and a reduction in the amount of waste. We found no increase in complications or difference in functional results between the two routes [12].

During the COVID period, streamlining the care pathway also enabled us to continue to offer care to patients without delaying treatment. It is also a valuable therapeutic option for cardiovascular patients, as their anticoagulant treatment can be pursued without modification or suspension, as well as for diabetic patients, as no preoperative fasting is required.

Take-Home Messages

Indication

Patient with surgery indications for carpal tunnel

Contraindication

Patients with cysts or external compression or any other indication for open surgery.

Surgical Technique

(a) WALANT anesthesia is done with 20 CC.
(b) The safe zone is drawn from the proximal flexion crease. At the wrist to the Kaplan line. On the medial side the ulnar nerve and artery are located and on the radial side the median nerve and its branches.
(c) Ultrasound is used to assess the position of the safe zone.
(d) The entry point is found with a needle; it should be located at the proximal wrist flexion crease.
(e) Open the skin with a knife with a 0.5 cm incision.
(f) The kemis is passed under ultrasound to control that the lower blade is under the ligament on a transverse view. Then the section is done under ultrasound control on a longitudinal view.
(g) The procedure is done until the ligament is cut.
(h) Control the release with a Halstead forceps on a transverse view.

Postoperative care

(i) Dressing for 48 h is essential to avoid hematoma.
(j) Free use of the hand is authorized immediately.

Conclusion

Ultrasound release of the carpal tunnel is feasible and reproducible with this mini-invasive technique. The recovery allows a quick return to daily activities.

Bibliography

1. Padua L, Cuccagna C, Giovannini S, Coraci D, Pelosi L, Loreti C, Bernabei R, Hobson-Webb LD. Carpal tunnel syndrome: updated evidence and new questions. Lancet Neurol. 2023;22(3):255–67. https://doi.org/10.1016/S1474-4422(22)00432-X. Epub 2022 Dec 13. PMID: 36525982.
2. Zamborsky R, Kokavec M, Simko L, Bohac M. Carpal tunnel syndrome: symptoms, causes and treatment options. Literature Review. Ortop Traumatol Rehabil. 2017;19(1):1–8. https://doi.org/10.5604/15093492.1232629. PMID: 28436376.
3. Seror P. Sonography and electrodiagnosis in carpal tunnel syndrome diagnosis, an analysis of the literature. Eur J Radiol. 2008;67(1):146–52. https://doi.org/10.1016/j.ejrad.2007.06.017. Epub 2007 Jul 31. PMID: 17669612.
4. Henry BM, Zwinczewska H, Roy J, Vikse J, Ramakrishnan PK, Walocha JA, Tomaszewski KA. The prevalence of anatomical variations of the median nerve in the carpal tunnel: a systematic review and meta-analysis. PLoS One. 2015;10(8):e0136477. https://doi.org/10.1371/journal.pone.0136477. Erratum in: PLoS One. 2015;10(9):e0138300. PMID: 26305098; PMCID: PMC4549253.
5. Moran L, Royuela A, de Vargas AP, Lopez A, Cepeda Y, Martinelli G. Carpal tunnel syndrome: diagnostic usefulness of ultrasound measurement of the median nerve area and quantitative elastographic measurement of the median nerve stiffness. J Ultrasound Med. 2020;39(2):331–9. https://doi.org/10.1002/jum.15111. Epub 2019 Aug 18. PMID: 31423615.
6. Orhurhu V, Orman S, Peck J, Urits I, Orhurhu MS, Jones MR, Manchikanti L, Kaye AD, Odonkor C, Hirji S, Cornett EM, Imani F, Varrassi G, Viswanath O. Carpal tunnel release surgery- a systematic review of open and endoscopic approaches. Anesth Pain Med. 2020;10(6):e112291. https://doi.org/10.5812/aapm.112291. PMID: 34150584; PMCID: PMC8207842.
7. Larsen MB, Sørensen AI, Crone KL, Weis T, Boeckstyns ME. Carpal tunnel release: a randomized comparison of three surgical methods. J Hand Surg Eur. 2013;38(6):646–50. https://doi.org/10.1177/1753193412475247. Epub 2013 Jan 22. PMID: 23340761.
8. Apard T, Candelier G. Surgical ultrasound-guided carpal tunnel release. Hand Surg Rehabil. 2017;36(5):333–7. https://doi.org/10.1016/j.hansur.2017.05.005. Epub 2017 Aug 16. PMID: 28822671.
9. Kazmers NH, Presson AP, Xu Y, Howenstein A, Tyser AR. Cost implications of varying the surgical technique, surgical setting, and anesthesia type for carpal tunnel release surgery. J Hand Surg Am. 2018;43(11):971–977.e1. https://doi.org/10.1016/j.jhsa.2018.03.051. Epub 2018 May 18. PMID: 29784549; PMCID: PMC6218304.

10. Leblanc MR, Lalonde DH, Thoma A, Bell M, Wells N, Allen M, Chang P, McKee D, Lalonde J. Is main operating room sterility really necessary in carpal tunnel surgery? A multicenter prospective study of minor procedure room field sterility surgery. Hand (N Y). 2011;6(1):60–3. https://doi.org/10.1007/s11552-010-9301-9. Epub 2010 Nov 18. PMID: 22379440; PMCID: PMC3041895.
11. Lalonde DH. "hole-in-one" local anesthesia for wide-awake carpal tunnel surgery. Plast Reconstr Surg. 2010;126(5):1642–4. https://doi.org/10.1097/PRS.0b013e3181f1c0ef. PMID: 21042120.
12. Moscato L, Helmi A, Kouyoumdjian P, Lalonde D, Mares O. The impact of WALANT anesthesia and office-based settings on patient satisfaction after carpal tunnel release: a patient reported outcome study. Orthop Traumatol Surg Res. 2023;109(3):103134. https://doi.org/10.1016/j.otsr.2021.103134. Epub 2021 Oct 29. PMID: 34715390.

Ultrasound-Guided Carpal Tunnel Release: The Retrograde Technique

9

Thomas Apard and Jules Descamps

9.1 Introduction

There are several methods to perform carpal tunnel release, including open carpal tunnel release, endoscopic carpal tunnel release, and ultrasound-guided carpal tunnel release (USCTR). USCTR is a minimally invasive technique where ultrasound imaging is used to guide the procedure, offering the potential for reduced recovery times and complications, while seeing the ulnar artery and median nerve.

In 1997, Nakamichi and Tachibana [1], orthopedic surgeons from Tokyo, published the first ultrasonographically assisted carpal tunnel release, later popularized by Rojo-Manaute [2], Rajeswaran [3], Petrover [4], and Apard [5]. A systematic review by Chou et al. [6] highlighted the potential effectiveness and safety of USCTR. Out of 1772 USCTR cases across 20 studies, a major complication was reported in only 1 patient (suspected compartment syndrome), and minor complications were noted in 24 patients. Many studies reported significant improvements in patient outcomes, with some noting these as early as the first week post-procedure.

T. Apard (✉)
Ultrasound Guided Hand Surgery Center, Versailles, France

J. Descamps
Department of Orthopedics and Trauma Surgery at Lariboisière Hospital, Paris, France

9.2 Personal Technique

Following the WALANT technique for anesthesia, as described by Lalonde et al. [7], 20 mL of the premixed saline (50%) and lidocaine 1% with epinephrine (45% and bicarbonate 8.4% (5%) has been injected with a 27G needle under the skin of the palm (and not in the carpal tunnel). The goal is to assess the anesthesia from the distal forearm (just above the radiocarpal joint seen under ultrasound) to the end of the carpal tunnel.

The hand was washed three times according to the antiseptic protocol. All the procedure was carried out with sterile gloves, sterile ultrasound cover, and gel in an interventional room or operating room.

An ultrasound is carried out so as to locate the safe zone between the ulnar artery and the median nerve as described by Nakamichi et al. [1] As a result, two parallel lines were drawn on the palm. The position of the vascular arch was also located to define the distal frontier of the safe zone. WALANT liquid created an anechoic area above the ligament, which improved its visualization ultrasonographically.

A 2 mm incision of the skin using a 19-gauge needle was performed between the two lines, which allows a hook blade to be placed under the junction of the antebrachial fascia and the flexor retinaculum. We used the needle to perforate the fascia in order to simplify the introduction of the device. The hook was steadily advanced under

O. Marès et al. (eds.), *Ultrasound-Guided Limb Surgery*,
https://doi.org/10.1007/978-3-031-88679-9_9

the ligament with continuous ultrasound monitoring (transversal and longitudinal views), until it reaches a few millimeters beyond it, before the vascular arch, and transected in a retrograde manner.

Before cutting the ligament, the surgeon had to be sure the hook was between the ulnar artery and the median nerve in transversal views and placed before the palmar arch artery in longitudinal view (Doppler mode could be helpful if needed).

Each step is described in Figs. 9.1, 9.2, 9.3, 9.4, 9.5, and 9.6.

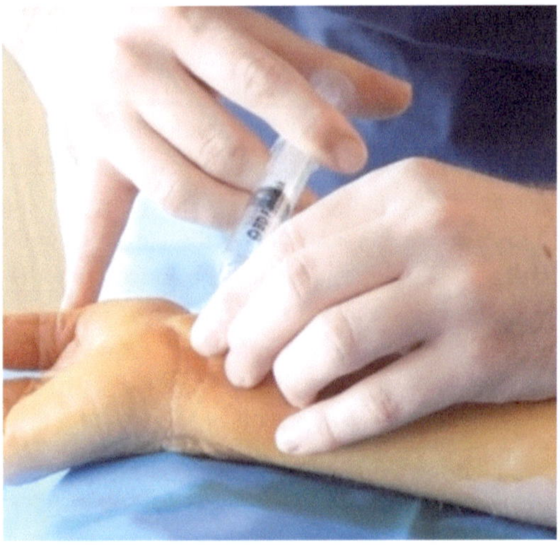

Fig. 9.1 Injection of local anesthesia

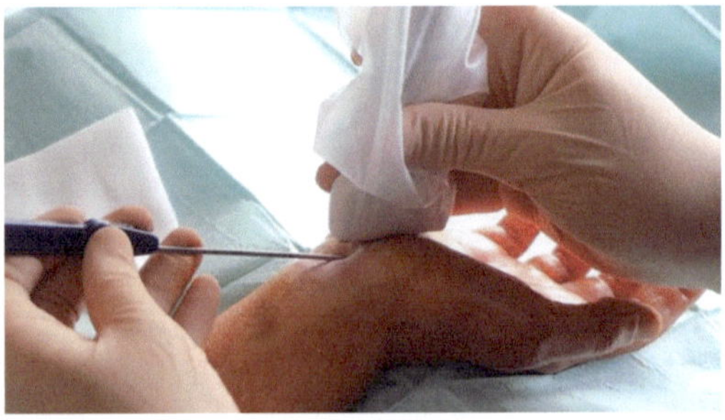

Fig. 9.2 Introduction of the hook

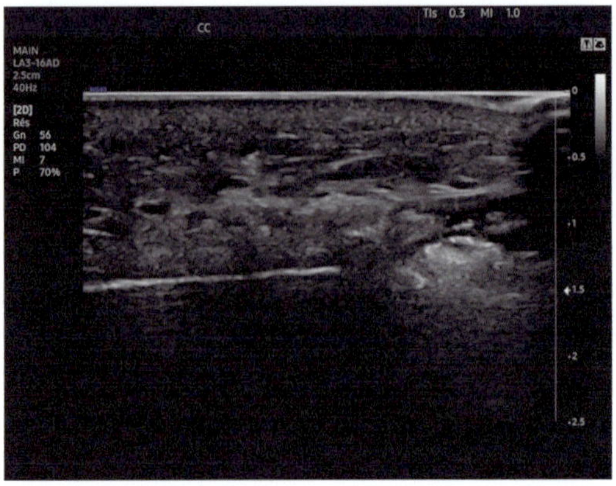

Fig. 9.3 Longitudinal view of the hook in the carpal tunnel

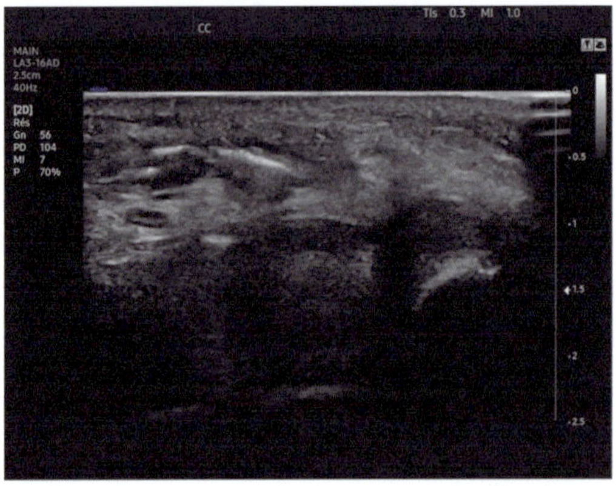

Fig. 9.4 Transverse view of the hook between the ulnar artery and the median nerve

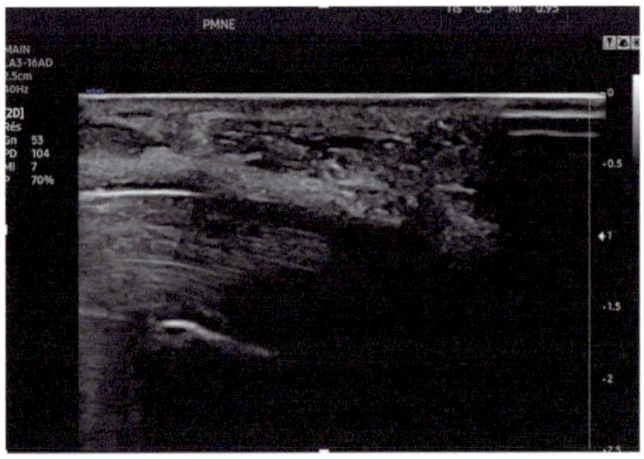

Fig. 9.5 Section of the ligament (longitudinal view)

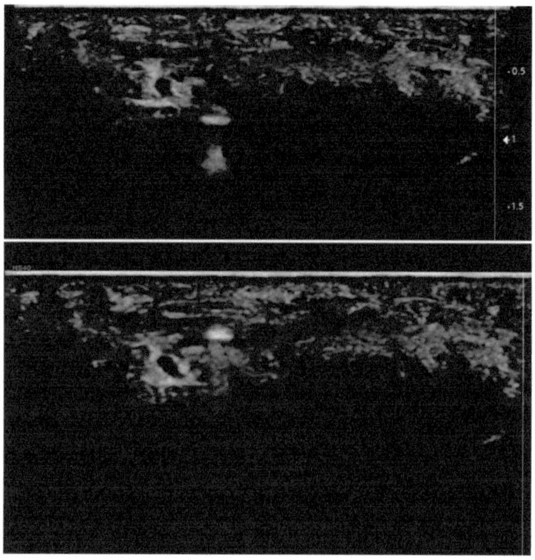

Fig. 9.6 Control of the complete release with the device passing through the ligament in transversal view. See the hook (horizontal white line) between the ulnar artery (on the left side) and the median nerve (on the right side)

9.3 Experience

Retrograde USCTR from November 2017 to May 2023 has been analyzed utilizing a natural language processing (NLP) model, specifically the DeepDocs SAS solution, for data extraction from clinical notes.

The study reviewed 816 retrograde USCTR procedures performed on 690 patients, 226 men (32.8%) and 464 women (67.2%). The mean age was 62 ± 16 years (range, 18–98). Among the patients, 17% were identified as smokers. Additionally, specific medical conditions were noted, 62 diabetes (9%), and 104 patients on anticoagulant/antiaggregant medications (15.1%).

Complications were systematically monitored and analyzed using the NLP model from clinical notes, focusing on various postoperative outcomes such as bleeding, hematoma, pillar pain, and numbness. This comprehensive approach allowed for a detailed assessment of the procedure's safety profile.

9.3.1 Outcomes

The primary outcome of this study was the disappearance of paresthesia, defined as the complete resolution of paresthesia symptoms following USCTR. Secondary outcomes included the presence or absence of pain, the subjective strength, and overall patient satisfaction. These outcomes were dichotomously recorded as either present or absent. The evaluation of the procedure's safety showed a low complication rate among the 816 USCTR procedures, with only 0.7% experiencing complications (6 patients in total, and 3 of those procedures had more than one complication). No conversion to open carpal tunnel release was needed. Hematomas were observed in six cases. These instances of hematoma resolved spontaneously without the need for further medical intervention. A single case reported a high pain syndrome on the day following the procedure, necessitating pain management including morphine and Lyrica, alongside a hospitalization period of 4 days. Two cases of ulnar hypoesthesia were documented, and one patient experienced postoperative stiffness. Notably, there were no reported infections following the USCTR procedures.

This study corroborates the effectiveness and safety of USCTR in the management of carpal tunnel syndrome, evidenced by significant improvements in paresthesia, pain, and strength, alongside high patient satisfaction rates. The low incidence of complications further supports USCTR as a viable, minimally invasive treatment option. Future research, ideally incorporating prospective designs and control groups, is warranted to validate these findings further and explore the procedure's long-term outcomes.

Bibliography

1. Nakamichi K, Tachibana S. Ultrasonographically assisted carpal tunnel release. J Hand Surg Am. 1997;22(5):853–62. https://doi.org/10.1016/S0363-5023(97)80081-0.

2. Rojo-Manaute JM, Capa-Grasa A, Chana-Rodríguez F, et al. Ultra-minimally invasive ultrasound-guided carpal tunnel release: a randomized clinical trial. J Ultrasound Med. 2016;35(6):1149–57. https://doi.org/10.7863/ultra.15.07001.
3. Rajeswaran G, Healy J, Lee J. Percutaneous release procedures: trigger finger and carpal tunnel. Semin Musculoskelet Radiol. 2016;20(05):432–40. https://doi.org/10.1055/s-0036-1594283.
4. Petrover D, Silvera J, De Baere T, Vigan M, Hakimé A. Percutaneous ultrasound-guided carpal tunnel release: study upon clinical efficacy and safety. Cardiovasc Intervent Radiol. 2017;40(4):568–75. https://doi.org/10.1007/s00270-016-1545-5.
5. Apard T, Candelier G. Surgical ultrasound-guided carpal tunnel release. Hand Surg Rehabil. 2017;36(5):333–7. https://doi.org/10.1016/j.hansur.2017.05.005.
6. Chou RC, Robinson DM, Homer S. Ultrasound-guided percutaneous carpal tunnel release: a systematic review. PM&R. 2023;15(3):363–79. https://doi.org/10.1002/pmrj.12801.
7. Lalonde D. Minimally invasive anesthesia in wide awake hand surgery. Hand Clin. 2014;30(1):1–6. https://doi.org/10.1016/j.hcl.2013.08.015.

10 De Quervain's Disease

Francisco Javier Ferreira

10.1 Introduction

De Quervain's disease (DQD), also known as De Quervain's tenosynovitis, is a painful condition that affects the tendons of the first dorsal compartment (FDC), similar to the one seen with trigger fingers. The tendons become inflamed and result in pain, swelling, and difficulty in performing everyday actions.

It was first described in 1895 by a Swiss surgeon named Fritz de Quervain [1], and it remains a common cause of wrist pain.

DQD is characterized by thickening and myxoid degeneration of the tendon sheath in the first dorsal compartment (FDC) of the wrist [2].

The FDC of the wrist is a complex anatomical structure that houses several anatomical features, including the extensor pollicis brevis (EPB) tendon, the abductor pollicis longus (APL) tendon, and the superficial branch of the radial nerve, among others (Fig. 10.1). The extensor retinaculum at the FDC is a thick band of connective tissue that wraps around the wrist to hold the tendons in place. The retinaculum acts as a pulley, redirecting the tendon's direction of pull and reducing the degree of friction caused by movement. The floor of the FDC is the radial styloid process, and surgical or traumatic changes at this point can develop DQD.

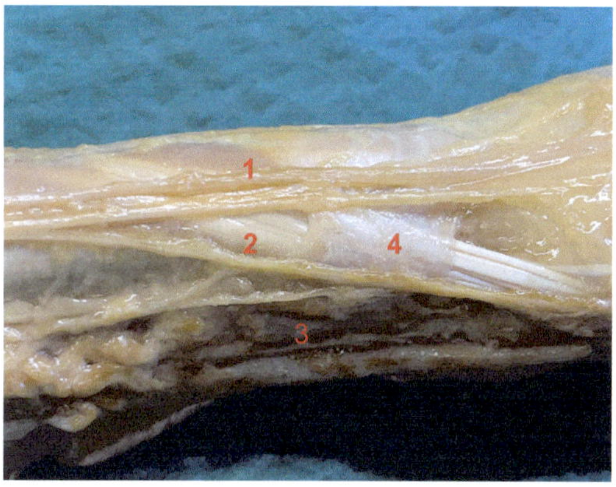

Fig. 10.1 Nerve anatomy around the first dorsal compartment. (1) Main dorsal branch of the radial nerve; (2) Lateral dorsal digital branch of the superficial radial nerve; (3) Lateral cutaneous nerve communications to the lateral dorsal digital branch; (4) First dorsal compartment

Many anatomical variations of the tendons have been described, but the most common and surgically relevant variant is the presence of separate tendon sheaths that are divided by a septum [3].

Supplementary Information The online version contains supplementary material available at https://doi.org/10.1007/978-3-031-88679-9_10.

F. J. Ferreira (✉)
Hospital Universitario San Rafael, Madrid, Spain

International Chair of Musculoskeletal Ultrasound, UCAM, Murcia, Spain
e-mail: javierferreira@drjavierferreira.com

O. Marès et al. (eds.), *Ultrasound-Guided Limb Surgery*,
https://doi.org/10.1007/978-3-031-88679-9_10

DQD disease is usually caused by overuse of the wrist and thumb or repetitive motions that cause the tendons to rub against the walls of the fibro-osseous tunnel. Certain occupations or hobbies that require frequent repetitive movements of the thumb and wrist may increase the risk of developing DQD [4].

10.2 Diagnosis

Diagnosis of DQD is based on patient's clinic history and physical examination. Finkelstein and Eichhoff tests are commonly used in clinical practice to diagnose DQD. The Finkelstein test involves the examiner firmly holding the patient's thumb with one hand and applying firm traction longitudinally and slight ulnar deviation to the wrist with the other hand, while the Eichhoff test requires the patient to oppose the thumb into the palm and clench their fingers while ulnar deviation is applied passively by the examiner. Recently the wrist hyperflexion and abduction of the thumb test (WHAT) has been advocated. During WHAT, the patient is asked to actively hyperflex the wrist and abduct their thumb as the examiner's index finger provides counterpressure, which will produce pain if DQD is present.

Radiographs are only helpful to rule out bony pathologies if we suspect previous trauma at the distal radius.

However, the use of ultrasound (US) has greatly helped us to correctly assess the structures involved in De Quervain's disease and identify the underlying pathogenesis [5], being able to make more precise therapeutic indications.

US is an effective diagnostic tool in the early detection of the disease. It allows for the proper identification of swollen tendons and can detect any tears or inflammation that may exist. It also has proven efficacy detecting the presence or absence of septum between APL and EPB that may aid in decreasing the incidence of post-treatment complications and regression of symptoms [5].

Unlike X-rays and MRIs, ultrasound is noninvasive and relatively inexpensive.

The ultrasound diagnosis for De Quervain's disease can reveal thickening or swelling of the tendons, or the retinaculum involved, which is indicative of the condition. The presence of fluid accumulation can also be detected through ultrasound.

Additionally, ultrasound can identify scar tissue or adhesions, which may have developed because of previous injuries or surgeries.

Ultrasonography also plays a critical role, not only in diagnosis but also in guiding local steroid injections and monitoring changes in the tendon sheath post-treatment.

10.3 Treatment

As with other orthopedic pathologies, nonoperative treatment should be indicated first, including immobilization, nonsteroidal anti-inflammatory drugs (NSAID), and corticosteroid injections [6]. US-guided injections have proved in several studies great rates of success [7, 8].

Although corticosteroid injections have shown a good success rate in the treatment of De Quervain's disease, there are several important complications described in the literature that can affect this result such as subdermal fat atrophy and necrosis, skin hypopigmentation, infection, post-injection flare, and radial nerve neuritis.

10.3.1 Surgical Management

Surgical release of the FDC is indicated when conservative treatment is unsuccessful.

Open release of the FDC has remained the standard surgical procedure since its description.

However, open release has known risks that can make the procedure fail such as hypertrophic and painful scarring, tendon instability, and injuries to the radial sensory nerve (RSN).

Despite the excellent outcomes of open release, in an attempt to improve the results in the short-term avoiding the complications seen in traditional surgery, minimally invasive techniques such as endoscopic or percutaneous release have been developed.

Although endoscopic FDC release has been shown to be effective, an increased procedure cost, longer operative time, and a long learning curve had been advocated as drawbacks.

Percutaneous release studies have shown good clinical results obtained despite partial release of the FDC revealed on cadaveric studies.

Ultrasound-guided release is a promising technique that has shown positive results in treating De Quervain's tenosynovitis, with few clinical studies published to date, all of them using a retrograde release technique (Table 10.1).

This technique uses ultrasound imaging to guide the surgeon, allowing for precise localization of the affected area and targeted delivery of treatment. It is a minimally invasive procedure that can be done on an outpatient basis, reducing the risk of complications associated with surgery such as bleeding or infection allowing for a quicker recovery time, with a very good level of cost efficiency, compared to open surgery, obtaining favorable results in more than 90% of cases [9, 10]. Because ultrasound-guided release of the first extensor compartment of the wrist is a highly precise and technically demanding procedure, it should be done by skilled hand surgeons who have experience with the open technique and with ultrasound-guided procedures.

10.3.2 Personal Technique

Candidates for ultrasound-guided percutaneous release would be those diagnosed with De Quervain's disease, without response to conservative treatment.

10.3.2.1 Prerequisites

A previous ultrasound study should be carried out with a linear, high-frequency probe (20 MHz desirable) for assessing the nerve structures, especially the radial sensory nerve since it emerges between the tendons of the brachioradialis muscle and extensor carpi radialis longus, in the so-called Wartenberg arch, and the first branch of this, the lateral dorsal digital branch to the thumb (LDDBT), as well as the terminal branches of the cutaneous lateral antebrachial nerve (Video 1). The LDDBT is especially relevant because it has close relation to the ventral portion of the FDC [11]. The location of the cephalic vein, which is in intimate relationship with the radial sensory nerve, is also important.

Only when we have a clear neurovascular pathway along the FDC, we will indicate the ultrasound-guided procedure.

Finally, we must assess the tendon structures of the first compartment and the presence of a septum, according to Hiranuma's classification. The latter is very important since the existence of a septum that separates the EPB from the APL forces us to double open the compartment and therefore makes surgery more difficult.

10.3.2.2 Setup (Fig. 10.2)

Surgery is performed under wide awake local anesthesia with no tourniquet (WALANT). A 10 ml of 1% lidocaine with 1:100.000 epinephrine buffered with 1 ml of 8.4% sodium bicarbonate is injected under the skin 3 cm proximal to the radial styloid if the nerve anatomy is favorable.

We prepare the surgical field with two small sterile drapes, one of them with a hole. Surgeon is equipped with sterile gown (optional) and gloves.

The skin is cleaned with chlorhexidine.

Table 10.1 De Quervain's tenosynovitis release case studies published (10/2023)

Author	Year	Study	Technique
Peck and Ely	2013	Case report	Retrograde
Lapegue et al.	2018	Prospective case study	Retrograde
Coldberg and Henderson	2019	Case report	Retrograde
Croutzet et al.	2019	Prospective case study	Retrograde
Shen et al.	2023	Controlled clinical trial	Retrograde
Beidleman et al.	2023	Retrospective case study	Retrograde

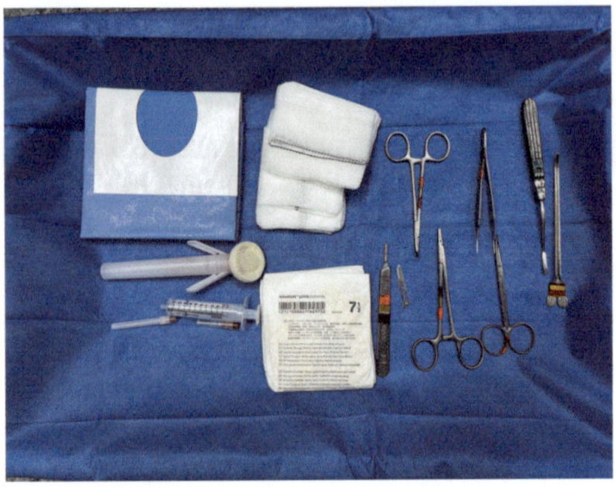

Fig. 10.2 Operating room setup

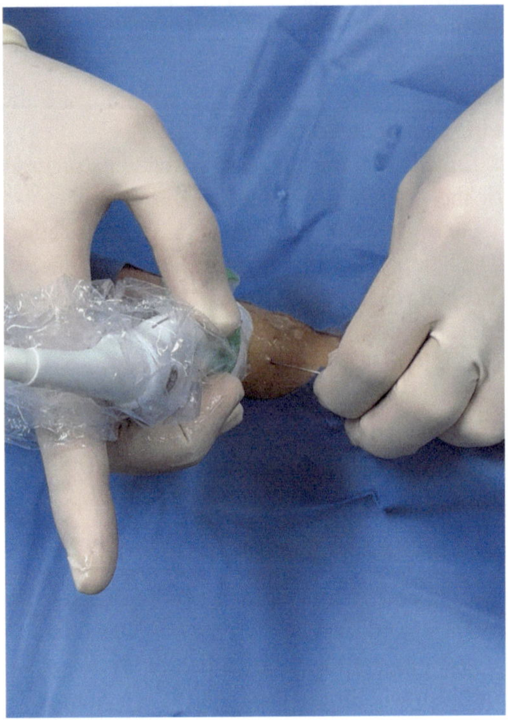

Fig. 10.3 Proximal incision (portal) location

The US probe is introduced in a sterile cover and sterile gel or chlorhexidine is used between the skin and the probe to avoid air interference.

10.3.2.3 Surgery (Video 2)

A 25G needle is introduced under US guidance about 3 cm proximal to the radial styloid tip (Fig. 10.3). Once proper location is achieved, a small transverse incision of 1–2 mm is made. A blunt dissector is introduced between the extensor retinaculum and the fat tissue to assure that vascular and neural structures are freed. Next, the cutting device is introduced into the proximal wound and the FDC is liberated from proximal to distal, in its dorsoulnar corner just on top of EPB. If there is a septum, the action should be repeated changing slightly the cutting device direction, shifting to a more volar position over APL.

Finally, under ultrasound control, it is checked with a forceps mosquito inside the FDC that the pulley has been released.

The closure of the surgical wound is not performed, covering it with a small dressing.

10.3.2.4 Postoperative Care

Wound home care instructions are provided.

The patients must perform tendon gliding exercises of the thumb and wrist. They can perform daily living activities without restriction normally after 72 h of surgery (after the end of the inflammatory phase of healing) but avoiding overuse during the first 3 weeks (proliferative phase).

Painkillers are prescribed for postoperative pain, especially the first 2 or 3 days. (Video 3)

10.4 Experience

Between June 2022 and December 2023, our institution conducted a total of 34 ultrasound-guided procedures on patients diagnosed with De Quervain's disease. We treated 32 patients, two of whom had bilateral symptoms. The average age of the patients was 40.2 years (ranging from 33 to 56). Visual analog scale for pain improved from 7.4 to 1.1, and quick-Dash score improves from 55 to 9,4. There were no major complications related with the procedure, although we recorded three minor complications: ecchymosis in two patients, first extensor compartment tenderness in two patients, and transient radial nerve numbness in one patient.

All patients returned to work at 6 weeks, highlighting the use of ultrasound-guided minimally invasive surgery in active population.

10.5 Conclusion

Ultrasound-guided WALANT surgery for De Quervain syndrome is a feasible and reliable procedure in good conditions. Ultrasound guidance allows to free all the septum of the De Quervain compartment in a safe manner.

Take-Home Messages

Indication

Patient with surgery indications for De Quervain release after failure of medical treatment

Contraindication

Patients that need open surgery:

Neuroma, ganglion, or cyst at De Quervain's level

Surgical Technique

(a) Local anesthesia with 10 ml of 1% lidocaine with 1:100.000 epinephrine buffered with 1 ml of 8.4% sodium bicarbonate.
(b) Control the radial sensitive branch position with an US transverse view and make an entry point with a 25G needle distal to its crossing over the compartment
(c) Transverse skin portal is made; blunt dissection of the subcutaneous tissue.
(d) Access the tendon compartment and release the pulley form proximal to distal.
(e) Release both compartments (EPB and APL) when a septum is present.

Postoperative care

Pressure dressing for 24 h.
No mobility restriction

References

1. de Quervain F. On a form of chronic tendovaginitis by Dr. Fritz de Quervain in la Chaux-de-Fonds. 1895. Am J Orthop (Belle Mead, NJ). 1997;26:641–4.
2. Clarke MT, Lyall HA, Grant JW, Matthewson MH. The histopathology of de Quervain's disease. J Hand Surg. 1998;23:732–4.
3. Bonczar M, et al. Anatomical variations in the first dorsal compartment of the wrist: meta-analysis. Folia Morphol (Warsz). 2022;82:766. https://doi.org/10.5603/fm.a2022.0081.
4. Ranney D, Wells R, Moore A. Upper limb musculoskeletal disorders in highly repetitive industries: precise anatomical physical findings. Ergonomics. 1995;38:1408–23.
5. Nagaoka M, Matsuzaki H, Suzuki T. Ultrasonographic examination of de Quervain's disease. J Orthop Sci. 2000;5:96–9.
6. Abi-Rafeh J, Kazan R, Safran T, Thibaudeau S. Conservative management of de Quervain Stenosing tenosynovitis: review and presentation of treatment algorithm. Plast Reconstr Surg. 2020;146:105–26.
7. Shin YH, Choi SW, Kim JK. Prospective randomized comparison of ultrasonography-guided and blind corticosteroid injection for de Quervain's disease. Orthop Traumatol Surg Res. 2020;106:301–6.
8. Kume K, et al. In de Quervain's with a separate EPB compartment, ultrasound-guided steroid injection is more effective than a clinical injection technique: a prospective open-label study. J Hand Surg Eur. 2012;37:523–7.
9. Beidleman MB, Colberg RE, Beason DP, Fleisig GS. A retrospective case series study on a minimally invasive ultrasound-guided first dorsal compartment release technique for refractory De Quervain tenosynovitis. Am J Phys Med Rehab. 2023;102:235–40.
10. Croutzet P, et al. Ultrasound-guided de Quervain's tendon release, feasibility, and first outcomes. J Wrist Surg. 2019;08:513–9.
11. Gurses IA, Coskun O, Gayretli O, Kale A, Ozturk A. The relationship of the superficial radial nerve and its branch to the thumb to the first extensor compartment. J Hand Surg. 2014;39:480–3.

11 Ultrasound-Guided Osteosynthesis of Distal Radius Fractures

Jean Michel Cognet and Olivier Mares

11.1 Introduction

Assessing the reduction of a distal radius or finger fracture and the subsequent implant positioning typically requires an intraoperative checking using fluoroscopy. Fluoroscopy requires protective measures because of ionizing radiation. The risk level varies based on the patient, duration of exposure, and repetitive nature of certain procedures. In several countries, fluoroscopy use also requires an accreditation that must be renewed every 3 years through training.

Ultrasonography (US) is a non-invasive image modality that is devoid of radiation risk, both for the patient and surgeon. US imaging can help us with the diagnosis of occult fractures and the evaluation of fracture reduction. The costs of purchasing and maintaining US systems have greatly decreased in recent years, and no radiation protective measures are required during use. We have combined this diagnostic ability with an assessment of the fixation of distal radius, metacarpal, and phalangeal fractures.

11.2 Equipment Needed

We currently use a Samsung system (HS 40) with a standard high-frequency probe (3–16 MHz) and a "hockey stick" high-frequency probe (17–18 MHz). Although it is possible to use a lower-frequency probe (4–12 MHz), the image quality will be lower but still acceptable for checking distal radius and finger fractures (Fig. 11.1).

Because the probe is not sterile, we use protective sleeves such as the ones used for arthroscopy. We recommend using an inner sleeve (provided with the single-use kit) and combining it with an arthroscopy sleeve (Fig. 11.2). Sterile gel is placed on the probe before applying the first sleeve, and then the second sleeve is used to cover the entire length of the probe's cable (Figs. 11.3, 11.4, and 11.5).

J. M. Cognet
Médipole, Bezannes, France

O. Mares (✉)
Department of Traumatology and Orthopedic Surgery, University Hospital Nîmes, Nîmes, France
e-mail: olol@gmail.es

O. Marès et al. (eds.), *Ultrasound-Guided Limb Surgery*,
https://doi.org/10.1007/978-3-031-88679-9_11

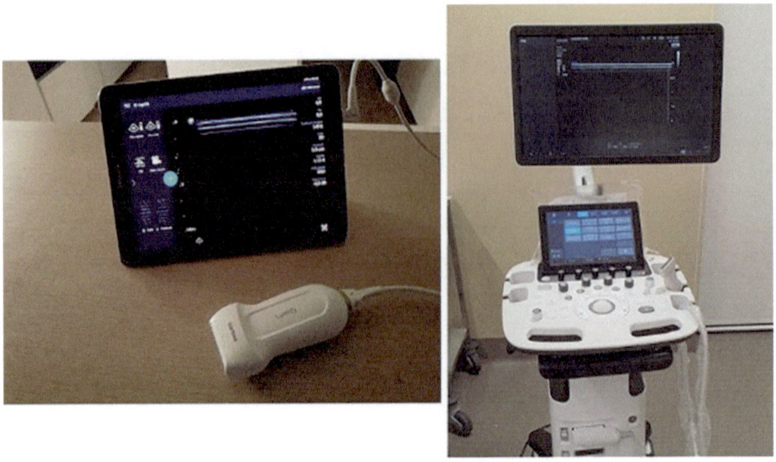

Fig. 11.1 A Philips® 4 to 12 MHz probe coupled with an Android tablet (*left*) and a SAMSUNG® HS 40 US system with 3 to 16 MHz probe (*right*)

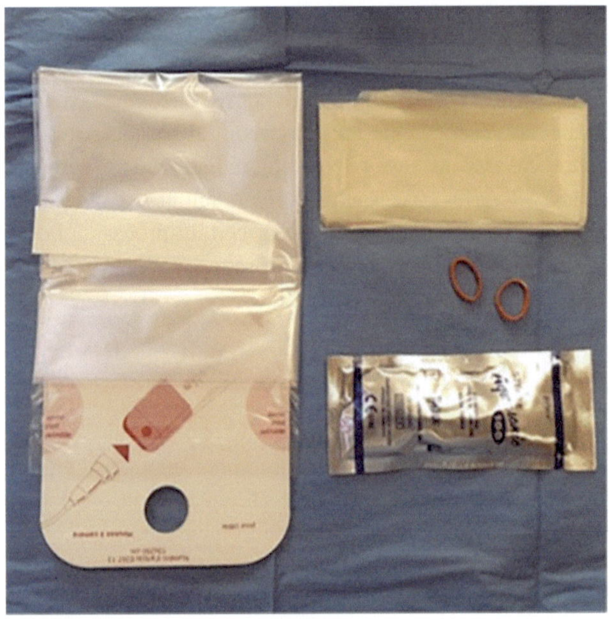

Fig. 11.2 Arthroscopy sleeve (*left*) and sleeve for US unit, elastics, and gel pocket (center from top to bottom)

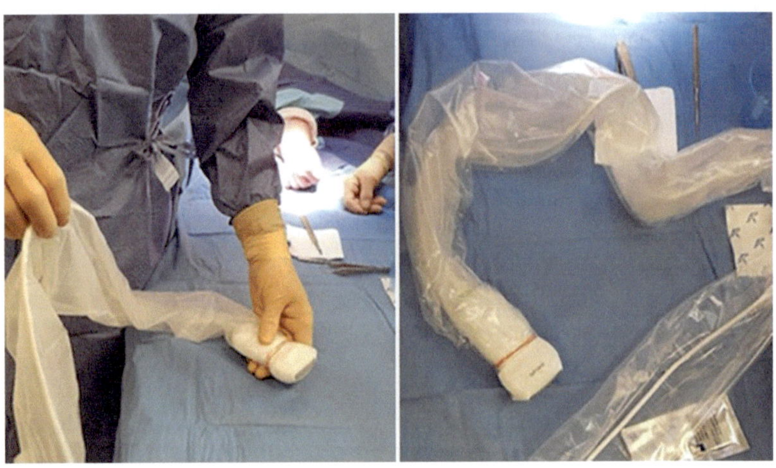

Fig. 11.3 Probe covered by an US sleeve (*left*) with an additional longer arthroscopy sleeve (*right*) that can cover the entire length of the cable

11.3 Technique

The patient is positioned supine, with a tourniquet at the base of the arm and the arm on an arm board; fluoroscopy system is placed facing the surgeon. The US probe rests on the operating table, and the device is located at the end of the arm board (see Figs. 11.4 and 11.5).

The gain is typically set at 60 and the depth at 3.5 cm for distal radius fractures and 1.5 cm from phalangeal/metacarpal fractures. Many systems allow a user's preferred settings to be stored so they can be reused each time.

11.3.1 Distal Radius Fractures

The procedure involves three steps, irrespective of the type of fixation:

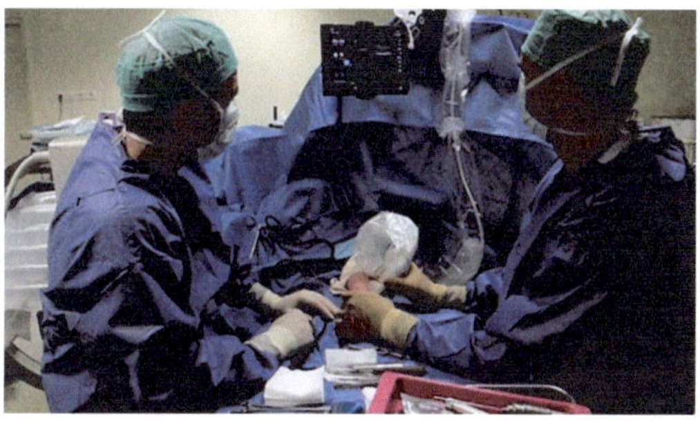

Fig. 11.4 Operating room setup; the surgeon manipulates the probe, with the screen on the right beside the patient and the surgical assistant standing across from them

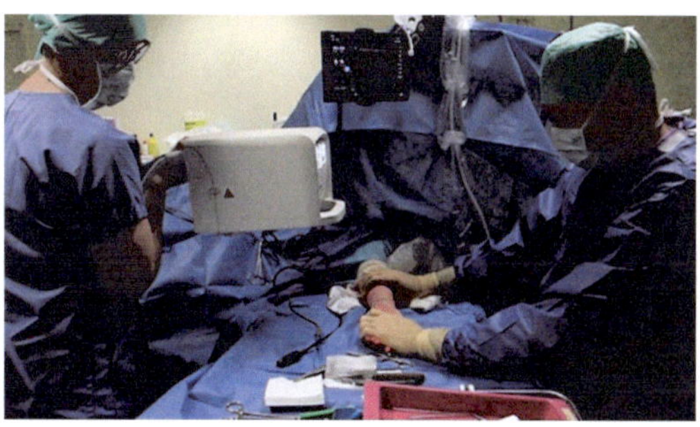

Fig. 11.5 Fluoroscopy can be paired with US when needed

11.3.1.1 Step 1: Ultrasonography Detection of the Fracture Lines and Comparison with Preoperative Radiographs

An initial scan is performed to locate the fracture site and detect any changes in the anatomic landmarks (Fig. 11.6):

Distal radioulnar joint on a transverse view (a)
Lister's tubercle on a transverse view (b)
Dorsal cortex of radius on a transverse view (c)
Anterior curvature of radius until the watershed line on a sagittal view (d)
Posterior cortex of distal radius on sagittal view (e)

The main landmarks are the anterior and posterior cortex of the distal radius. On a fracture with posterior tilt, the dorsal cortex is always modified and clearly visible. Loss of the anterior curvature is sometimes harder to detect on a dorsally displaced fracture. Transverse views of Lister tubercle and the diaphysis display an interesting elevator effect when done dynamically: sweeping the US probe over the dorsal side of the distal radius from proximal to distal will identify gradual elevation of the diaphysis up to Lister tubercle. In case of a dorsally displaced fracture, there is a sudden change in diameter from the diaphysis to the metaphysis of the radius; in some instances, there will be a double contour when the bones overlap.

Other structures are easy to pinpoint such as the pronator quadratus and the surrounding nerves, arteries, and tendons.

11.3.1.2 Step 2: Reduction and Stabilization of Fracture Site

The US step does not alter the fixation technique in any way. We typically use a locking plate designed specifically for distal radius fractures. However, although the fracture site is stabilized by the plate, we used the PY technique to reduce the fracture site. Pinning can be done either before the plate is applied, after using US as a reference, or simply based on the preoperative

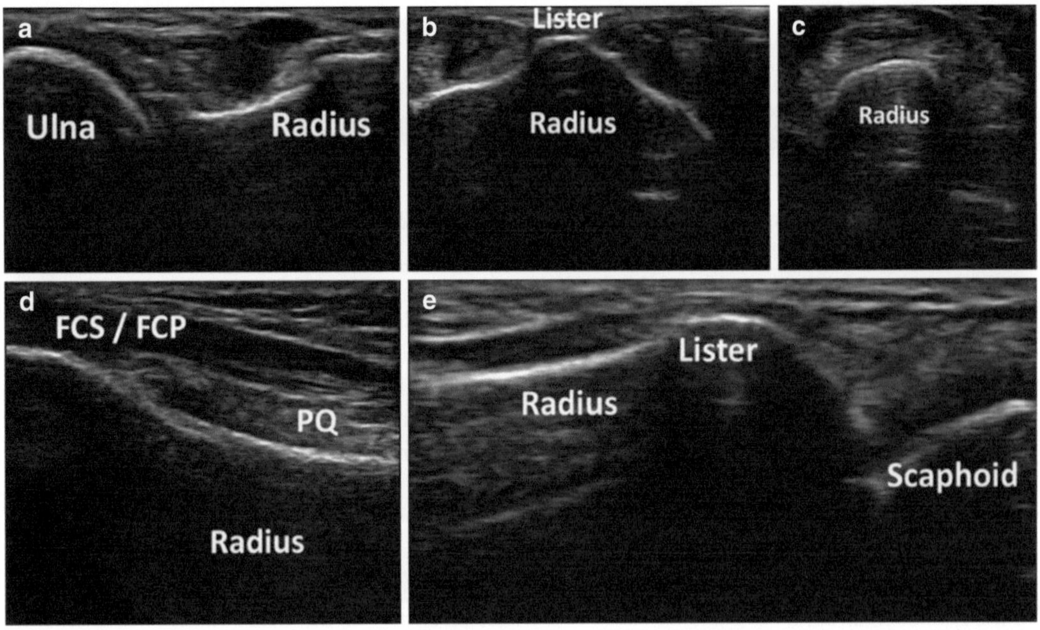

Fig. 11.6 Anatomic landmarks for the wrist on US: distal radioulnar joint on a transverse view (**a**), Lister tubercle on a transverse view (**b**), dorsal cortex of radius on a transverse view (**c**), anterior curvature of radius up to the watershed line on a sagittal view (**d**), posterior cortex of distal radius on a sagittal view (**e**)

radiographs. It is done by hand, without a motorized handpiece.

If the initial reduction is done first with K-wires, US images are then taken to check the reduction. The bone topography of the anterior cortex is visible on US with much better definition than on images generated by fluoroscopy (Fig. 11.7). When the displacement is mainly posterior without a break in the anterior cortex, US imaging assesses the reduction of the posterior cortex, which is also clearly visible (Fig. 11.8).

In certain cases, excessive reduction can be observed on US even though it cannot be seen on fluoroscopy (Fig. 11.9).

The volar plate can be implanted through a volar approach. A visual check of the fracture site is done to confirm the US images. The locking plate is set in its anterior position and held in place by a non-locking screw placed in the oval slot. The plate's position is adjusted relative to the watershed line and the lateral edges of the radius shaft; the preferred location is on the ulnar aspect of the radial diaphysis.

Another US image is taken at this point to verify anatomic landmarks avoiding excessive reduction. Once the plate is in place, it is more difficult to see the anterior cortex on US; thus, the check revolves around Lister tubercle and the radial side of the distal radius. At this point, we look for dorsal cortical breach of the first screw.

If there is a large displacement, US is used to identify the median nerve, evaluate its integrity, and look for impingement by a bone splinter (Figs. 11.10 and 11.11); this is especially valuable when the patient presents with paresthesia in the territory of the median nerve.

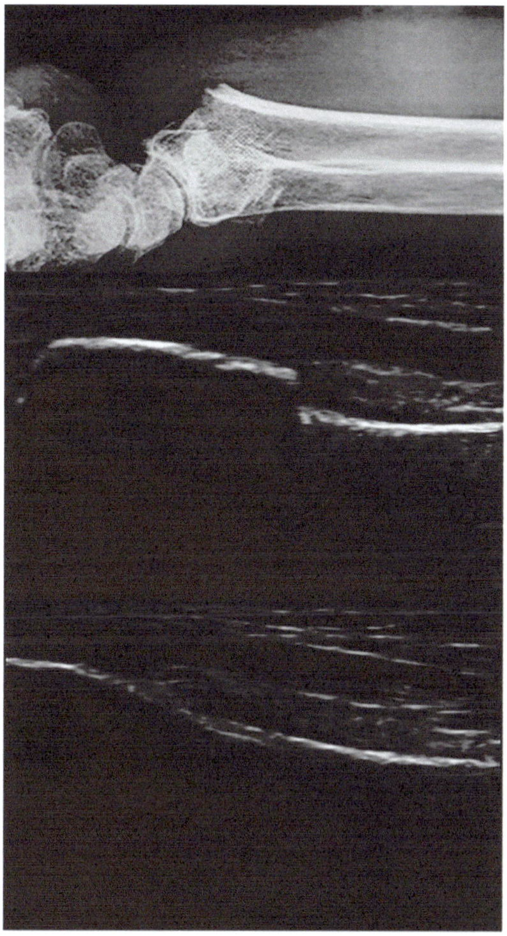

Fig. 11.7 US view of the reduction of the anterior cortex

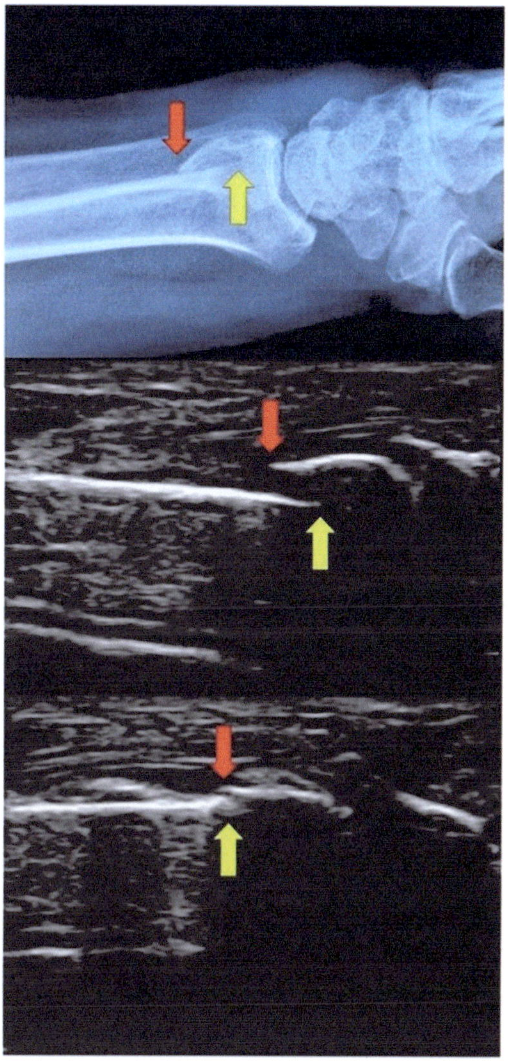

Fig. 11.8 US view of the reduction of the posterior cortex of the distal radius

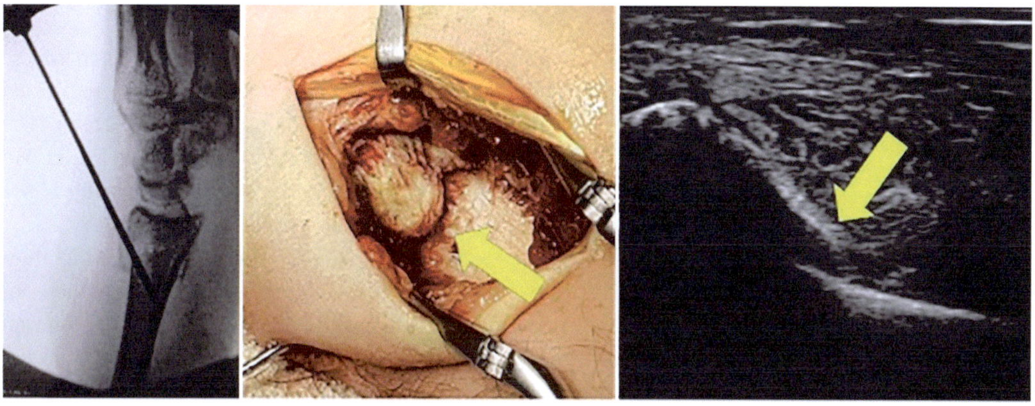

Fig. 11.9 This anterior over-reduction is not visible on fluoroscopy but was detected with US; note the good match between the US image and the intraoperative appearance

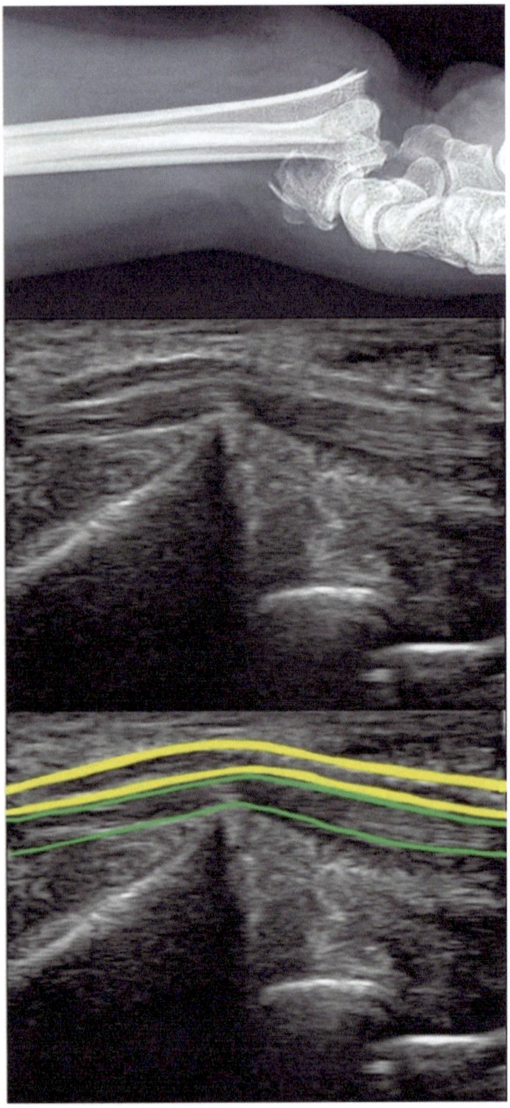

Fig. 11.10 Extra-articular distal radius fracture with large displacement; the patient described having paresthesia in the median nerve territory. Sagittal US view before and after reduction showing the location of the flexor tendons (green) and the median nerve (yellow) relative to the fracture site: despite the large displacement, we can see that the median nerve is still protected by the flexor tendons

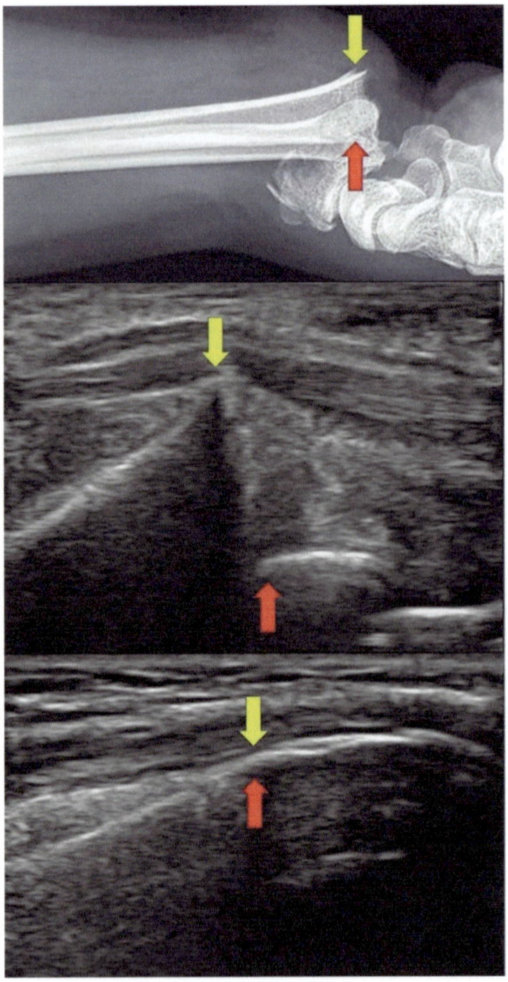

Fig. 11.11 Ultrasonography verification of reduction based on anterior cortex of distal radius; red arrow corresponds to proximal limit of distal fragment; yellow arrow corresponds to distal limit of proximal fragment. When the two arrows are lined up, the fracture is reduced

11.3.1.3 Step 3: Final Fixation

If the surgeon is not certain whether the plate is in the correct position (too distal) or is concerned about a screw protruding inside the joint, a K-wire is pushed into the drilled hole and its exit point checked with US. Once the epiphyseal screws are in place, the surgeon moves the wrist to ensure there is no impingement with the implanted device (intra-articular projection of screw). The distal radioulnar joint also needs to be tested. We look at the dorsal cortex of the distal radius to see if a screw is sticking out (Fig. 11.12).

In early cases, we recommend pairing fluoroscopy with US at each step to confirm the fracture's reduction and the plate's correct positioning. One should start with simple, extra-articular fractures (e.g., Pouteau/Colles). Later on, a surgeon can progress to using this tech-

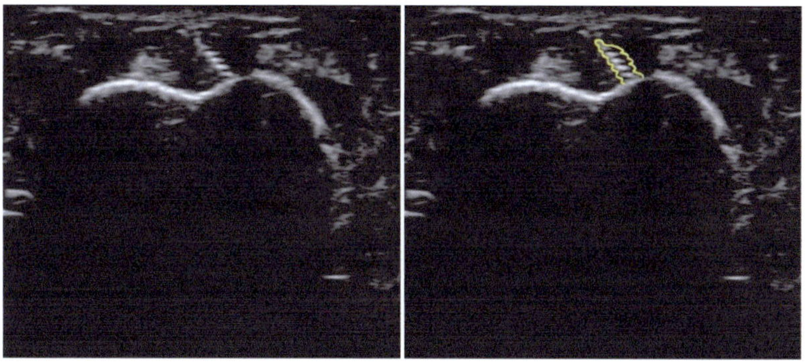

Fig. 11.12 Frontal view of the radial metaphysis where a screw protrudes beyond the cortex

nique with intra-articular fractures as long as it is combined with arthroscopy assessment. In fact, it is impossible to view the intra-articular step off or subsidence if the fracture occurred in the central area of the scaphoid's or lunate's articular fossa.

11.4 Discussion

Intraoperative verification of fracture fixation requires the use of a X-ray device in the operating room, providing images of the fracture reduction and implants. However, radiographs are harmful to the human body, with known increased risks of skin cancer, especially in hand surgery, but also of thyroid cancer and cataracts [1–3]. In recent years, the introduction of mini C-arm systems designed for the extremities has reduced the risks related to ionizing radiation but has not eliminated them [4]. Finding an alternative to X-rays during fracture fixation would be a positive step both for patients and surgical team.

There are currently no published articles that reported the possibility of doing US-guided distal radius fracture fixation. The existing studies describe verifying the reduction of distal radius fractures [5–7]. Conversely, studies have been done to compare fixation of a metacarpal facture with either fluoroscopy or US guidance [8, 9].

Ang and colleagues reported their results of closed wrist fracture reduction on an emergency basis. By generating US images, the number of manipulations was reduced, and the reduction improved.

In 2014, Kodama and colleagues compared 43 patients with distal radius fracture that were reduced by US guidance to 57 patients who had their fracture reduced manually with or without fluoroscopy assistance. Success of the reduction was the same in both groups.

More recently, Lau and colleagues evaluated the contribution of US to the diagnosis and verification of reduction in patients with distal radius fracture. They also determined how the person doing the US (radiologist or not) affected the result. Here again, US yielded results equal to that of radiography, independent of the operator.

Pediatricians have been using US to diagnose traumatic fractures for several years. The sensitivity of US is better than the sensitivity of radiographs for detecting fractures in children [10–13]. The specificity of US is better than the specificity of radiographs. Chen and Moore [9] found 14 false positives due to radiographs in a cohort of 110 children who had a nondisplaced fracture of both forearm bones.

In adults, US imaging is at the forefront when radiographs are not sufficient to make a diagnosis. This is the case for fatigue fractures where radiographs are normal at early stages, whereas US can reveal the changes needed to make a diagnosis [14]. Banal and colleagues [13] showed that the sensitivity of US was equal to that of MRI but that US was easier to schedule and cost substantially less. The availability of US and the miniaturization of the workstations have contributed to US being increasingly used in sports medicine [14]. A fracture could be diagnosed immediately after the injury occurs, even when there is no access to an X-ray machine.

Several investigators contend that US diagnosis of fractures should be expanded to all bone traumas. Its relevance is supported in situations where radiographs can be misleading, as in bone injuries in the emergency room [15].

However, US-guided plate fixation of a fracture has its challenges, with a good positioning of the plate on the radius and verification of screw trajectory and exit point.

For all the above, ultrasound is a tool that the orthopedic surgeon can use to facilitate fracture diagnosis and improve the quality of the per-operative reduction. The learning curve is fast for an experienced surgeon. The common use of ultrasound control for the management of distal radius fractures reduces ionizing radiation to the patient, surgeon, and staff. The quality of images produced by ultrasound and the association with artificial intelligence will improve the quality of trauma management in the future.

Take-Home Messages

Indication

Patient with surgical indication of an extra-articular distal radius fracture

Contraindication

Intra-articular fractures without an extra-articular component

Surgical Technique

(a) Circular control to evaluate the distal ulna and radius lesion.
(b) Control the median nerve position.
(c) After closed reduction assessment of the quality of the reduction and research of any entrapment of soft tissue.
(d) Final fixation of the fracture.
(e) Circular control to assess the quality of the reduction.
(f) If not good: modify until the best reduction is obtained.
(g) If good: assess any conflict between the hardware and the soft tissue.
(h) Repeat as necessary.

Postoperative care

(i) Pressure dressing for 24 h
(j) Immobilization of the type of fracture needed

11.5 Conclusion

Ultrasound control of distal fractures is a feasible solution. That allows control of both the quality of the bone reduction and assesses also the conflict of the soft tissue with the hardware.

Bibliography

1. Chambers JA, Long JN. Radiation injury and the hand surgeon. J Hand Surg Am. 2008;33(4):601–11.
2. Frazier TH, Richardson JB, Fabre VC, Callen JP. Fluoroscopy-induced chronic radiation skin injury: a disease perhaps often overlooked. Arch Dermatol. 2007;143(5):637–40.
3. Mastrangelo G, Fedeli U, Fadda E, Giovanazzi A, Scoizzato L, Saia B. Increased cancer risk among surgeons in an orthopaedic hospital. Occup Med (Oxford, England). 2005;55(6):498–500.
4. van Rappard JRM, Hummel WA, de Jong T, Moues CM. A comparison of image quality and radiation exposure between the mini C-arm and the standard C-arm. Hand (New York, NY). 2018:1558944718770210.
5. Shah CM, Sommerkamp TG. Fracture dislocation of the finger joints. J Hand Surg Am. 2014;39(4):792–802.
6. Kodama N, Takemura Y, Ueba H, Imai S, Matsusue Y. Ultrasound-assisted closed reduction of distal radius fractures. J Hand Surg Am. 2014;39(7):1287–94.
7. Lau BC, Robertson A, Motamedi D, Lee N. The validity and reliability of a pocket-sized ultrasound to diagnose distal radius fracture and assess quality of closed reduction. J Hand Surg Am. 2017;42(6):420–7.
8. Ko C, Baird M, Close M, Cassas KJ. The diagnostic accuracy of ultrasound in detecting distal radius fractures in a pediatric population. Clin J Sport Med. 2017;
9. Chen L, Kim Y, Moore CL. Diagnosis and guided reduction of forearm fractures in children using bedside ultrasound. Pediatr Emerg Care. 2007;23(8):528–31.
10. Chaar-Alvarez FM, Warkentine F, Cross K, Herr S, Paul RI. Bedside ultrasound diagnosis of nonangulated distal forearm fractures in the pediatric emergency department. Pediatr Emerg Care. 2011;27(11):1027–32.

11. Warkentine FH, Horowitz R, Pierce MC. The use of ultrasound to detect occult or unsuspected fractures in child abuse. Pediatr Emerg Care. 2014;30(1):43–6.
12. Fukushima Y, Ray J, Kraus E, Syrop IP, Fredericson M. A review and proposed rationale for the use of ultrasonography as a diagnostic modality in the identification of bone stress injuries. J Ultrasound Med. 2018.
13. Banal F, Gandjbakhch F, Foltz V, Goldcher A, Etchepare F, Rozenberg S, et al. Sensitivity and specificity of ultrasonography in early diagnosis of metatarsal bone stress fractures: a pilot study of 37 patients. J Rheumatol. 2009;36(8):1715–9.
14. Hoffman DF, Adams E, Bianchi S. Ultrasonography of fractures in sports medicine. Br J Sports Med. 2015;49(3):152–60.
15. Oguz AB, Polat O, Eneyli MG, Gulunay B, Eksioglu M, Gurler S. The efficiency of bedside ultrasonography in patients with wrist injury and comparison with other radiological imaging methods: a prospective study. Am J Emerg Med. 2017;35(6):855–9.
16. Bouillis J, Lallouet S, Ropars M. Echography-guided pinning for prevention of iatrogenic injuries to the radial nerve during fixation of extra-articular distal radius fracture: an anatomical study. J Wrist Surg. 2017;6(4):336–9.
17. Vosbikian MM, Ketonis C, Huang R, Ilyas AM. Optimal positioning for volar plate fixation of a distal radius fracture: determining the distal dorsal cortical distance. Orthop Clin North Am. 2016;47(1):235–44.
18. Imatani J, Akita K, Yamaguchi K, Shimizu H, Kondou H, Ozaki T. An anatomical study of the watershed line on the volar, distal aspect of the radius: implications for plate placement and avoidance of tendon ruptures. J Hand Surg Am. 2012;37(8):1550–4.
19. Obert L, Loisel F, Huard S, Rochet S, Lepage D, Leclerc G, et al. Plate fixation of distal radius fracture and related complications. Eur J Orthopaedic Surg Traumatol. 2015;25(3):457–64.
20. Gurbuz Y, Kucuk L, Gunay H, Ozaksar K, Sugun TS, Bilge O. Comparison of ultrasound and dorsal horizon radiographic view for the detection of dorsal screw penetration. Acta Orthop Traumatol Turc. 2017;51(6):448–50.
21. Vernet P, Durry A, Nicolau X, D'Ambrosio A, Collinet A, Botero Salazar S, et al. Detection of penetration of the dorsal cortex by epiphyseal screws of distal radius volar plates: anatomical study comparing ultrasound and fluoroscopy. Orthopaedics Traumatol Surg Res. 2017;103(6):911–3.

Part IV

Elbow

12 Epicondylitis

Olivier Marès, Jad Mansour, Sarah Pradel, and Pascal Kouyoumdjian

12.1 Introduction

Lateral epicondylitis (LE), also known as tennis elbow, is a painful condition that affects the common wrist extensor tendon at its insertion at the lateral epicondyle [1]. The prevailing opinion is that LE is a degenerative process, as the histology shows a tendinosis [2].

It is manifested by pain on the lateral side of the elbow, during the extension of the wrist and the formation of the fist. The first treatment is a conservative option with 90% of success, leaving about 10% of refractory cases for surgery [3]. Operative procedures for LE may be broadly grouped into three main categories: open, ultrasound-guided, and arthroscopic [4].

A new treatment system has been developed with US guidance for releasing the ECRB. This minimally invasive procedure using the Kemis® device (Newclip Technics) was originally designed for carpal ligament release [5].

This chapter introduces an innovative ultrasound-guided percutaneous method that uses a minimally invasive surgical knife. The "simplicity" of this technique ensures consistent complete release while minimizing complications. This is well aided by the real-time visualization by ultrasound guidance.

The shift from conventional open surgical methods to minimally invasive percutaneous and ultrasound-assisted techniques mark a significant advancement in treating epicondylitis. These methods not only are effective in relieving symptoms but also notably cut down on costs and surgery time and reduce potential risks. Additionally, they offer the benefit of a shorter postoperative recovery period.

A preoperative US examination is done. Preoperative scanning includes a longitudinal and transversal exploration to asses tendinosis, ruptures, and calcifications at ECRB/EDC junction.

All patients had previously undergone conservative treatment for at least 6 months. This included oral NSAIDs, injection of hydrocortisone, platelet-rich plasma (PRP), or shockwave therapy.

12.1.1 Diagnosis

The diagnosis of epicondylitis is primarily clinical. Patients report pain during extension of the wrist and the fingers. The pain can lead to impairment and adaptation to the work situation.

The discomfort and mechanical symptoms are localized at the lateral epicondyle.

O. Marès (✉) · S. Pradel · P. Kouyoumdjian
Department of Traumatology and Orthopedic Surgery, University Hospital Nîmes, Nîmes, France

J. Mansour
Division of Orthopedic Surgery and Sport Medicine, University of Toronto, Toronto, ON, Canada

O. Marès et al. (eds.), *Ultrasound-Guided Limb Surgery*,
https://doi.org/10.1007/978-3-031-88679-9_12

Patients may also experience increased stiffness, especially in the morning, and a progressive loss of forces of the extensor muscle. Palpation of the lateral elbow should research pain at the lateral epicondyle and try to exclude other possible diagnoses:

- Absence of an articular disk at the radiohumeral joint, related to pain at prono supination
- Absence of scratch collapse test at the posterior interosseus nerve at froshe's arcade
- Absence of posterolateral rotatory instability of the elbow

In addition to these clinical signs, the diagnosis can be supported by ultrasonography and MRI, which is particularly useful in visualizing the pathology at the tendon insertion. This imaging modality can confirm the diagnosis.

We usually rule out the other diagnoses mentioned before with US exploration:

12.2 US-Guided Surgical Technique

12.2.1 Setup

We use a US material linear probe (GE) in musculoskeletal mode at 13 MHz. A confirmatory US examination is performed before sterile preparation of the arm.

The patient is placed in the supine position, the affected arm on a hand table, and the elbow at 90° of flexion. The lateral aspect of the elbow is then prepped and sterilely draped in the usual fashion. Anesthesia is realized according to the protocol widely awake local anesthesia no tourniquet (WALANT) [6], with lidocaine plus epinephrine (Fig. 12.1).

A sterile US transducer sleeve and gel are used to ensure sterility of the US probe throughout the entirety of the procedure.

We start the procedure by first spotting the structures at risk: the lateral collateral ligament and the posterior lateral cutaneous nerve.

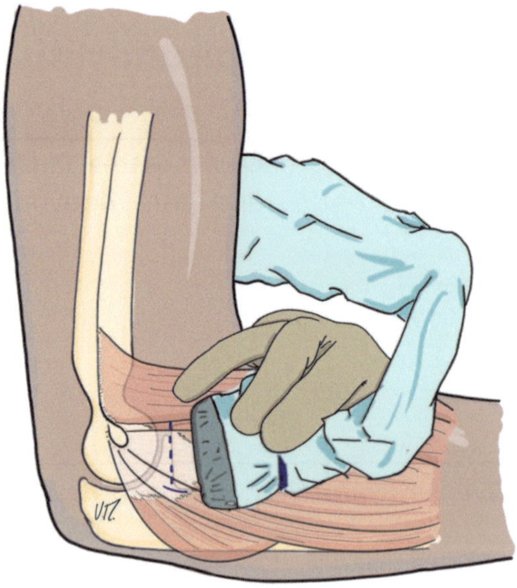

Fig. 12.1 View of the work zone

Then the junction between ECRB and EDC is identified in the coronal and frontal plane at a mean distance of 2 cm from the lateral epicondyle, just at the radial head level. The patient is asked to make an active extension of the wrist to visualize the fascia between ECRB and ECRL. This fascia is convex on the ECRB/EDC side during flexion of the wrist and shifts to concave during extension in the transverse view (Fig. 12.2a, b).

In a coronal view, a needle is passed beneath the ECRB from the lateral to the medial side to ensure the best entry point of the device to release the fascia (Fig. 12.3).

The skin is open on 0.5 cm and then smooth forceps are passed under the ECRB/EDC on the deep part of the tendon (Fig. 12.4). The supinator muscle is separated from the deep fascia of the ECRB. The Kemis® device is then inserted and during all procedures, the Kemis® device is under full control of US guidance.

The section starts from lateral to medial and the tendon is released and its aponeurosis. The aim is to release the fascia to obtain a large lengthening of the lateral fascia of the lateral muscles of the epicondyle (Fig. 12.5a, b).

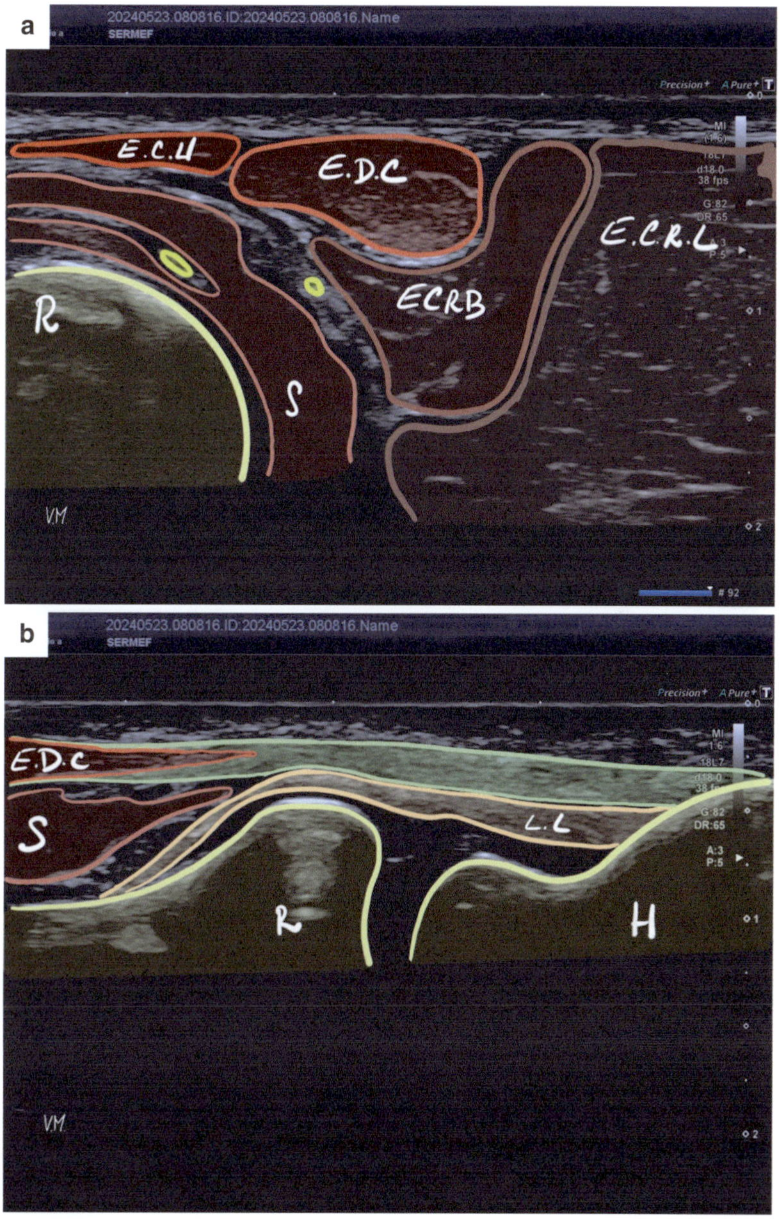

Fig. 12.2 (**a**) Ultrasound tranverse view of the lateral epicondyle. (**b**) Ultrasound longitudinal view of the lateral epicondyle

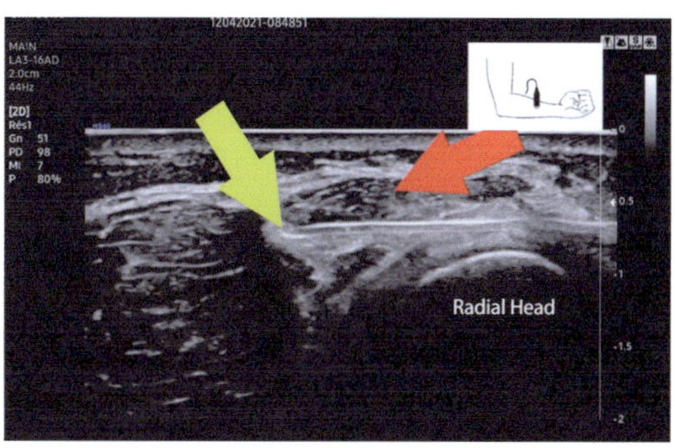

Fig. 12.3 US transverse of view of the needle

A transverse view with the Kemis® (Newclip Technics) knife during section at a distance of the supinator muscle

Smooth forceps are passed to be sure to have completely released the tendon on a transverse view.

A simple dressing with a bulky bandage is applied for 24 h. Then a simple dressing done by the patient is recommended. The delay for skin healing is 3 to 4 days. We never use stitches or glue.

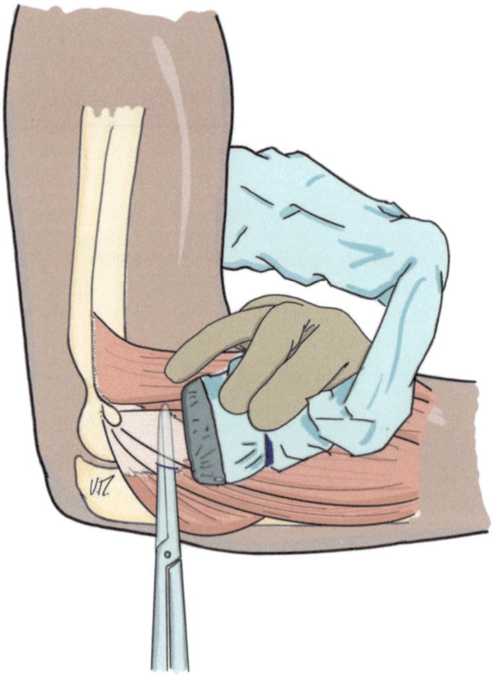

Fig. 12.4 View of the Halstead

12.3 Postoperative Care

The patient is informed that there will be postoperatively for 2/3 month a depression at the level of the fascia lengthening, which will disappear spontaneously with the healing process. The patient is asked to use his arms immediately after the procedure. We advocate no specific immobilization. Physiotherapy is initiated a few days after surgery. Heavy activities are encouraged after 8 weeks. Postoperative analgesia is realized with classic pain killer of level one with non-steroidal anti-inflammatory drugs (NSAIDs) for 1 week.

We have realized a case control between our first case of epicondylitis under ultrasound guidance compared to a comparable series of patients treated by arthroscopic.

All were assessed pre- and postoperatively using the Disabilities of the Arm, Shoulder, and Hand (DASH) score and the visual analog scale (VAS) pain score. Time to return to work, as well as complication rate, was reported.

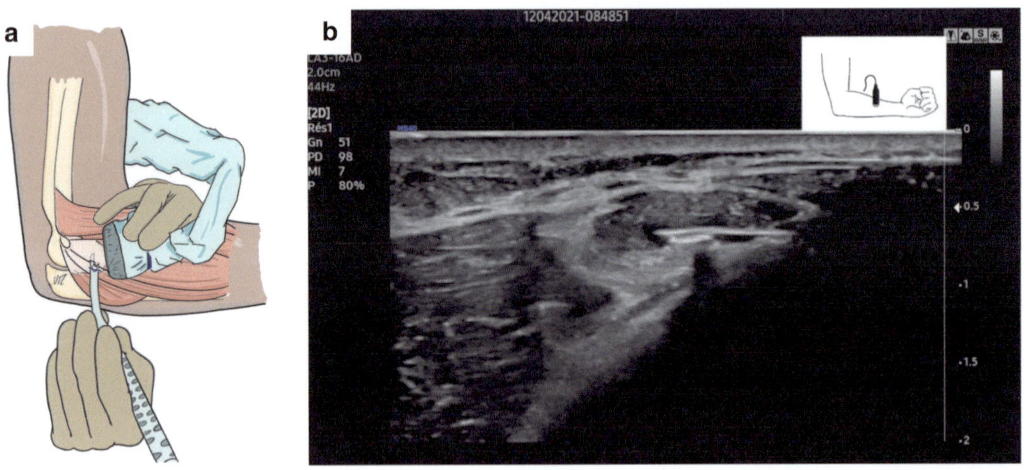

Fig. 12.5 (a) transverse view of the section. (b) ultrasound transverse view of the section

Postoperatively, patients were classified, according to their subjective satisfaction with surgery, as (1) satisfied, (2) partially satisfied, and (3) dissatisfied.

12.3.1 Experience

Eighteen patients, including 7 females and 11 males with a mean age at surgery of 50 years (range, 43–60), were operated on via mini-invasive procedure under US guidance, while the remaining 18, including 6 females and 12 males with a mean age at surgery of 48 years (range, 39–61), were subject of arthroscopic surgery, forming the control group.

The time frame is different because the US technique has been recently incorporated in the department.

All patients were engaged predominantly in manual work. The release was performed on the dominant side seven times in both groups. The mean follow-up time was 9 months (range, 6–13) for the US group and 39 months (range, 20–57) for the arthroscopic group. This difference was highly significant (p = 0.001) between the two groups.

For ultrasound-guided surgery, the mean DASH improved (p = 0.09), from 77.06 (range, 65.51–89.16) to 38.76 (range, 1.72–67.85). The mean VAS pain score also improved, from 8.63 (range, 6–10) to 3.25 (range, 0–8) with a mean decrease of 5.38 (range, 0–10) postoperatively (p = 0.92).

For arthroscopy, the mean DASH improved (p = 0.01) from 70.85 (range, 51.78–90.74) to 24.25 (range, 7.14–40.74), while the mean VAS pain score improved from 9.25 (range, 8–10) to 3.13 (range, 0–7), with a mean decrease of 6.13 (range, 3–9) postoperatively (p = 0.26). Only two patients in both groups were pain-free at the final follow-up that represents 25%.

The difference in DASH score improvement was insignificant between both groups (p = 0.20). This difference was also not significant in the VAS score decrease (p = 0.91).

There was no significant difference in mean time return to work among both groups, although it was faster for the US group with a mean time to return to work in 8 weeks compared to 14 weeks in the arthroscopic group (p = 0.11). Note that two patients in each group did not yet resume their functions.

Complex regional pain syndrome (CRPS) was the unique complication in both groups: with a rate of 12% in the US group compared to 25% with arthroscopic surgery. Nonetheless, the difference was not significant.

We had no infection nor dystrophic scars in either group.

There were 13 patients satisfied (75%) and 5 dissatisfied (25%) with US-guided technique, while 11 patients were satisfied (62.5%) and 7 patients were partially satisfied (37.5%) with the arthroscopic procedure. The difference was not significant between both techniques (p = 0.74).

The study showed that although all patients were engaged in manual tasks, the timeline for resumption to professional activities was shorter in the US group (8 weeks) than in the arthroscopic group (14 weeks) (p = 0.11).

The complication rates were inferior in the US group.

The present study provided promising outcomes with good tolerance among all patients within an office setting and slight evidence of equivalence in symptomatic and functional improvements compared to arthroscopic surgery, at least in short-term follow-up.

Take-Home Messages

Indication

Epicondylitis

Contraindication

Elbow lateral instability

Radial nerve compression

Intra articular disk

Surgical Technique

(a) Local anesthesia with 40 cc lidocaine + epinephrin 1%.
(b) Control common insertion of ECRB and EDC position with a US transverse view and make an entry point with a 27G needle at the level of the neck of the radial head.
(c) 3 mm skin incision with a 15-blade parallel.
(d) Subcutaneous dissection with an Halsted forceps. Pierce the fascia. Control the position of the instrument on a transverse and longitudinal view.
(e) Knife introduction. Verify on transverse and longitudinal view.
(f) Gently push the knife distally (holding your probe horizontally) to release the fascia as far as possible.
(g) Check the complete freeing of the fascia using a Halsted forceps.

Postoperative care

Pressure dressing for 24 h
No mobility restriction

Bibliography

1. Ahmad Z, Siddiqui N, Malik SS, Abdus-Samee M, Tytherleigh-Strong G, Rushton N. Lateral epicondylitis: A review of pathology and management. Bone Jt J. 2013;95 B(9):1158–64.
2. Regan W, Wold LE, Coonrad R, Morrey BF. Microscopic histopathology of chronic refractory lateral epicondylitis. Am J Sports Med. 1992;20(6):746–9.
3. Sevier TL, Wilson JK. Treating lateral epicondylitis, vol. 28. Sports Med. Springer; 1999. p. 375–80.
4. Lo MY, Safran MR. Surgical treatment of lateral epicondylitis: A systematic review. Clin Orthop Relat Res. 2007;463:98–106.
5. Mares O, Cognet JM, Apard T, Candelier G. Épicondylite latérale: nouvelle procédure sous contrôle échographique permettant de libérer le tendon de l'extenseur radial du carpe [abstract]. Hand Surg Rehabil. SFCM. 2019;38(6):451.
6. Lalonde D. Wide awake local anaesthesia no tourniquet technique (WALANT). BMC Proc BioMed Central Ltd. 2015;9(S3):A81.

13 Ultrasound-Guided Percutaneous Release of Ulnar Nerve at the Elbow

Bérénice Moutinot, Pascal Kouyoumdjian, and Olivier Marès

13.1 Introduction

Ulnar nerve compression is the second most common nerve entrapment syndrome of the upper extremity after carpal tunnel syndrome [1]. The annual incidence in France is about 21–25 cases/100,000 inhabitants [2]. The etiology is multifactorial. Male sex, local anatomy, and occupational activities are known to be risk factors [3].

The ulnar nerve is a sensory-motor nerve arising from C8-T1 roots. From proximal to distal, it gives branches to flexor carpi ulnaris, fourth and fifth flexor digitorum profundus, abductor digiti minimi, opponens digiti minimi, palmar interossei, dorsal interossei, third and fourth lumbricals, adductor pollicis, and the deep head of flexor pollicis brevis muscle. There are multiple potential sites of ulnar nerve compression at the elbow, mainly the arcade of Struthers, the medial intermuscular septum, the cubital tunnel retinaculum, Osborne's fascia, and Amadio and Beckenbaugh arcade. The two most frequent sites are the cubital tunnel retinaculum, which is the band between the medial epicondyle and the olecranon, and Osborne's fascia, which is the fusion of the aponeurotic fibers emanating from the two chiefs of the flexor carpi ulnaris (FCU) [4–7].

Despite a rich literature on the surgical options for ulnar tunnel syndrome, the optimal treatment remains controversial with no consensus on the ideal procedure.

13.2 Diagnosis

The diagnosis of ulnar nerve entrapment at the elbow is based on clinical signs and symptoms. Patients would typically complain of medial elbow pain with numbness and paresthesia in the medial side of the forearm and the two last digits. Symptoms could be present at night or daily especially during activities requiring prolonged elbow flexion as the cubital tunnel area decrease of 30–41% in this position. [8]

Loss of dexterity and strength could also be noticed with possible interossei atrophy. A pseudo-Tinel sign is often found at the compression site.

The diagnosis is primarily clinical as electrodiagnostic studies could be negative in early stage. However, electroneurogram remains the gold standard as it can specify myelin sheath and axon involvement. Ultrasound is also a useful diagnostic tool. It has the advantage of being able to observe anatomical variations such as the presence of an accessory muscle and to assess the stability of the nerve during flexion-extension movements of the elbow.

B. Moutinot
Centre Hospitalier de Genève, Geneva, Switzerland

P. Kouyoumdjian · O. Marès (✉)
Department of Traumatology and Orthopedic Surgery, University Hospital of Nîmes, Nîmes, France

O. Marès et al. (eds.), *Ultrasound-Guided Limb Surgery*,
https://doi.org/10.1007/978-3-031-88679-9_13

When an ulnar nerve entrapment at the elbow is suspected, several points need to be checked with the ultrasound.

13.2.1 The Size of the Nerve

The size cutoff point above which an ulnar nerve at the elbow is considered pathological is still open to debate. However, it is generally accepted that a size greater than 10 mm^2 is considered pathological [2]. A difference in caliber of more than 2 mm between the compression zone and the upstream zone is also recognized as abnormal. On a longitudinal view (obtained more easily with the elbow in extension), a pseudoneuroma can be seen proximal to the compression site.

13.2.2 The Aspect of the Nerve

With ischemia secondary to nerve compression, the classic honeycomb appearance of the nerve can change. The nerve will appear more hypoechogenic and undifferentiated. Intraneural hyperemia may sometimes be seen on color Doppler [7].

13.2.3 The Position of the Nerve

To determine whether the nerve is stable, simply hold the probe transversely between the medial epicondyle and the olecranon and progressively flex the elbow. If the nerve passes above the medial epicondyle, the latter is considered unstable. Checking whether the nerve is unstable is a prerequisite for percutaneous release, because if it is unstable, the patient will require transposition in addition to conventional neurolysis, and open surgery will therefore be preferred.

13.3 Treatment

The ideal treatment for ulnar nerve compression at the elbow remains controversial. Conservative treatment can be attempted in mild case without sensory or motor deficits by encouraging the patient to avoid prolonged elbow flexion or direct pressure on the ulnar nerve. Night rest splints with the elbow at 30° extension are also considered, but therapeutic adherence is limited due to the discomfort of wearing this type of splint and its effectiveness is debated [9].

13.3.1 Surgical Management

Despite a rich literature on the surgical options for ulnar tunnel syndrome, the optimal treatment remains controversial with no consensus on the ideal procedure. However, most studies report a faster recovery with less morbidity within situ decompression compared to neurolysis-transposition [10–13].

The release of the overlying tissues (arcade of Struthers) is a matter of debate. Some studies have reported that in situ neurolysis could concern only the cubital tunnel retinaculum and Osborne's fascia, justifying a miniaturization of the approach either with endoscopic techniques or "mini-open" [14, 15]. Those minimally invasive techniques reported good results with an optimized recovery time.

The controversy surrounding the need to release the fibers proximal to Osborne's fascia gave rise to the idea of a minimally invasive technique limited to the release of the cubital tunnel retinaculum and the flexor carpi ulnaris fibers under ultrasound guidance. The possibility to monitor the integrity of the ulnar nerve during the entire procedure makes this technique safe and effective with the advantage of eliminating the need for an arthroscopic tower.

Poujade et al. in 2014 and then Guo et al. in 2019 had already analyzed the feasibility of this technique with cadaveric studies. In both cases, the authors reported a complete release of the nerve on its portions around the elbow without iatrogenic injury [16, 17]. Compared with open surgery, percutaneous release using ultrasound guidance is a faster procedure with no increase in morbidity [18].

A parallel can be drawn between endoscopic procedure and ultrasound-guided percutaneous technique. Indeed, in both techniques, the skin incision is much smaller compared to an open approach and the dissection of the soft tissues is limited, which decrease the risk of perineural adhesion. Comparative series between endoscopic release and open in situ decompression shows similar results but faster recovery with the endoscopic technique [19, 20]. Time off work also seems to be reduced and patients return quicker to their daily activities [21].

13.3.2 Personal Technique

Candidates for ultrasound-guided percutaneous release of ulnar nerve at the elbow would be all patients with McGowan stage 1 or 2 ulnar nerve compression.

13.3.2.1 Prerequisites

Patients with a history of elbow fracture or a prior ulnar nerve surgery are not good candidates as perineural adhesion status makes percutaneous surgery difficult. Moreover, an instable nerve (checked clinically and by ultrasound) and a severe McGowan 3 nerve compression are also not good candidates for a percutaneous technique under ultrasound as they are better treated opened with an associated transposition.

13.3.2.2 Setup

This technique is performed as an outpatient procedure or office surgery under WALANT (Wide Awake Local Anesthesia and No Tourniquet) using a miniKemis® knife (NewClip Technics®, France) (Fig. 13.1). The patient is placed in prone position or laterally if external rotation of the shoulder is limited. The entire limb is included in the operating field. WALANT anesthesia requires a fluid volume of 20 cc consisting of 10 cc of 1% adrenalized xylocaine and 10 cc of saline. 15 cc are used for cutaneous anesthesia, and 5 cc are kept for deeper hydrodissection under ultrasound. The injection is performed with a 27-gauge needle. A high-frequency 9/16 MHz linear probe, protected by a sterile cover during the whole procedure, is mandatory.

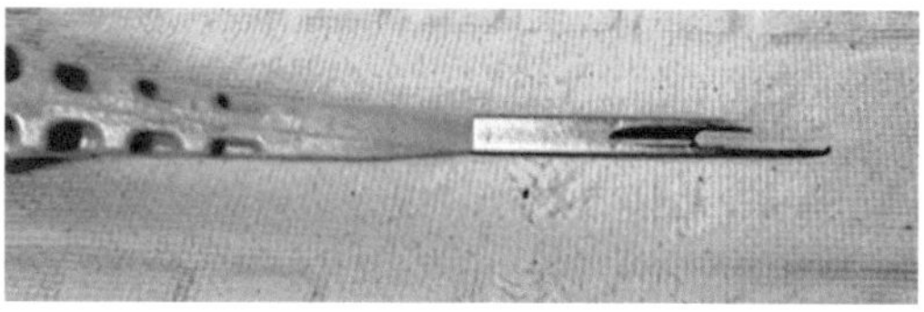

Fig. 13.1 miniKemis® knife (NewClip Technics®, France) with its mechanism of cutting

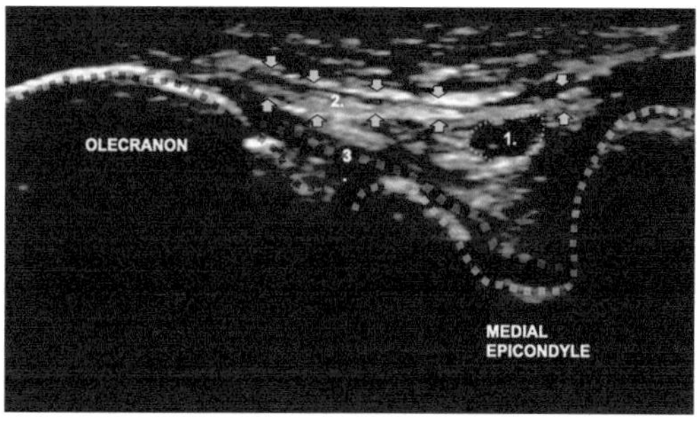

Fig. 13.2 Proximal transverse view at elbow level between olecranon and medial epicondyle: (1) Ulnar nerve, (2) (green arrows) cubital retinaculum, (3) medial collateral ligament

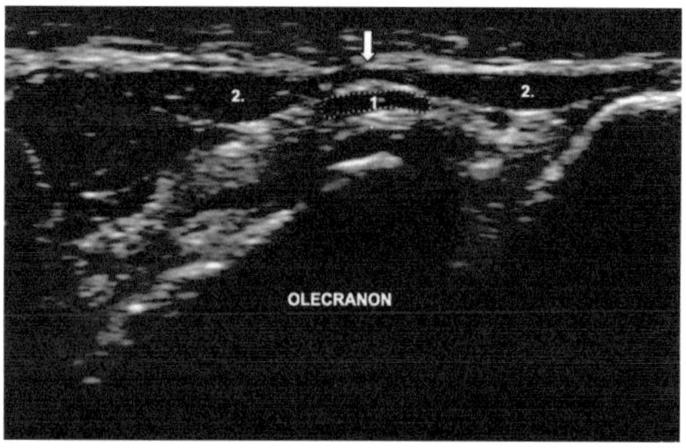

Fig. 13.3 Distal transverse view at the junction of the two heads of the flexor carpi ulnaris. (1) Ulnar nerve, (2) (dotted line) two heads of FCU, green arrows end of Osborne's fascia

13.3.2.3 Surgery

The elbow is positioned in slight flexion. The nerve is identified in its groove beyond the elbow joint in longitudinal and transverse views (Figs. 13.2 and 13.3). The proximal border of the cubital retinaculum is marked. The future entry point is then located on a transverse section with an intramuscular needle (Fig. 13.4). The objective is to obtain the best angle of approach with

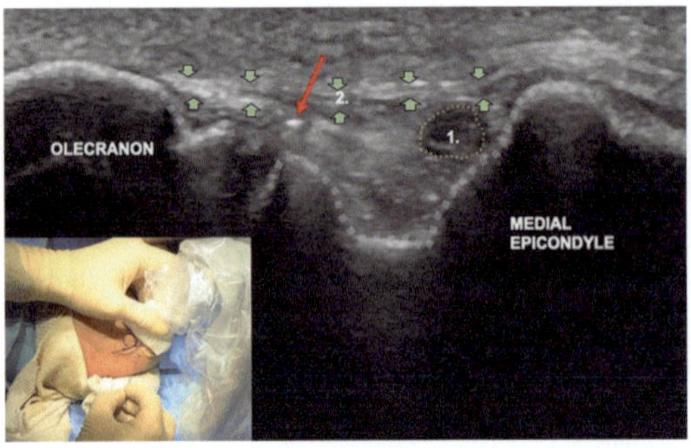

Fig. 13.4 Transverse view at elbow level between olecranon and medial epicondyle: (1) Ulnar nerve, (2) cubital retinaculum, red arrow: needle

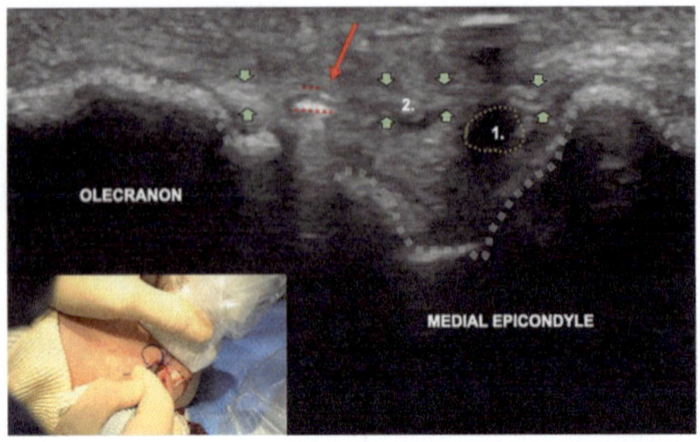

Fig. 13.5 Transverse view at elbow level between olecranon and medial epicondyle: (1) Ulnar nerve, (2) cubital retinaculum, red arrow: miniKemis (dotted lines: upper and lower blade)

the miniKemis® (New Clip), thus ensuring complete sectioning of the proximal fibers of the cubital retinaculum. A skin incision of less than 3 mm is made parallel to the skin with the N°15 blade scalpel proximal to the olecranon. A Halsted forceps is then introduced allowing dissection of the subcutaneous tissue without damaging any crossing branch of the medial antebrachial cutaneous nerve. The Halsted must pierce the retinaculum.

The miniKemis® knife is then introduced at the level of the skin incision. A transverse and longitudinal view are performed to verify the correct positioning of the knife. The distal tip must be under the arch of the FCU and outside the nerve (Fig. 13.5). The position of the nerve is continuously monitored during the procedure. When the knife is in place, the section of the arcade is performed by a section from proximal to distal with a longitudinal control view (Fig. 13.6). The complete section is then checked with a Halsted forceps on a transverse section, which should be able to move freely from the deep surface of the FCU to the skin. The section concerns only the cubital retinaculum and Osborne's fascia (Fig. 13.7). Neither Amadio and Beckenbaugh's arch nor Struthers' arch is released.

Ulnar nerve's stability is assessed by dynamic maneuver of flexion/extension of the elbow with an ultrasound control.

The wound is simply closed with Steri-strip® type adhesives.

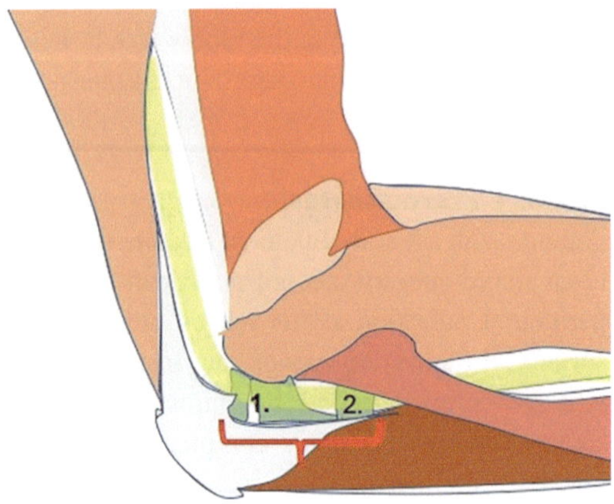

Fig. 13.6 Longitudinal view at the proximal forearm level: red dotted lines, miniKemis knife; green arrow, cubital retinaculum and Osborne's fascia

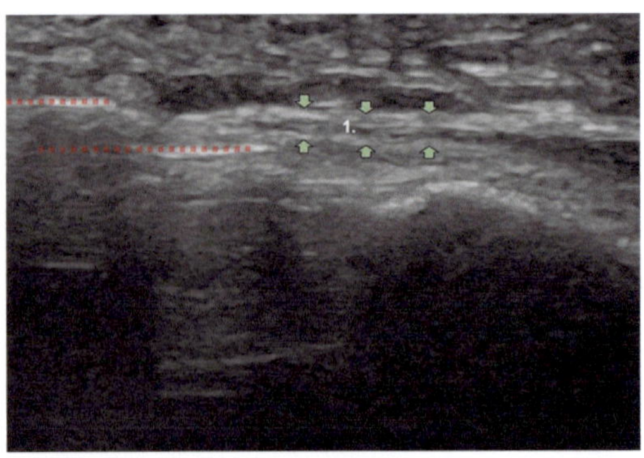

Fig. 13.7 Schematic elbow anatomy (medial view). (1) Cubital retinaculum, (2) Osborne's fascia

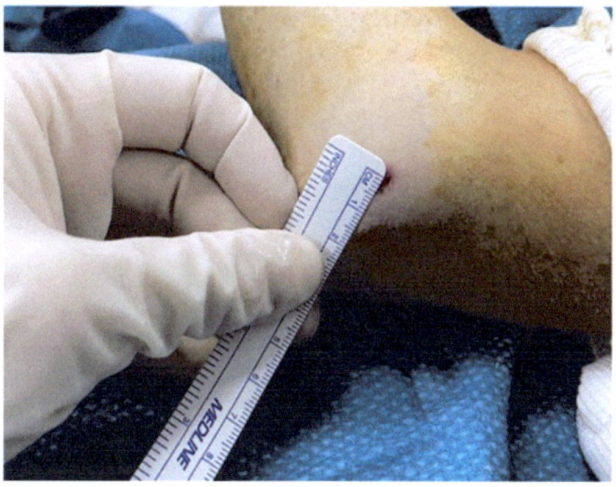

Fig. 13.8 Medial view of the elbow: final aspect of the scar

13.3.2.4 Postoperative Care

A pressure dressing for 24 h is applied. Level 1 painkillers are prescribed postoperatively. Wound home care instructions are provided because no nursing care is needed (Fig. 13.8). The patient is allowed to resume his or her activities immediately after the operation, avoiding the carrying of heavy loads for 15 days.

Take-Home Messages

Indication

McGowan 1–2 ulnar nerve compression.

Contraindication

Nerve instability

Disturbed local anatomy (history of elbow fracture, previous ulnar nerve neurolysis)

Surgical Technique

(a) Local anesthesia with 20 cc rapid epinephrin 1%
(b) Control ulnar nerve position with a US transverse view and make an entry point with a 27G needle proximal to the cubital tunnel retinaculum
(c) 3 mm skin incision with a 15-blade parallel to the skin
(d) Subcutaneous dissection with a Halsted forceps. Pierce the retinaculum. Control the position of the instrument on a transverse and longitudinal view
(e) Knife introduction. Verify on transverse and longitudinal view that only the lower blade is under the cubital retinaculum
(f) Gently push the knife distally (holding your probe horizontally)
(g) Check the complete freeing of the nerve using a Halsted forceps

Postoperative care

Pressure dressing for 24 h.
No mobility restriction

Bibliography

1. Mondelli M, Giannini F, Ballerini M, Ginanneschi F, Martorelli E. Incidence of ulnar neuropathy at the elbow in the province of Siena (Italy). J Neurol Sci. 2005;234(1–2):5–10. https://doi.org/10.1016/j.jns.2005.02.010.
2. Cambon-Binder A. Ulnar neuropathy at the elbow. Orthop Traumatol Surg Res. 2021;107(1S):102754. https://doi.org/10.1016/j.otsr.2020.102754.
3. Fernandez E, Pallini R, Lauretti L, Scogna A, La Marca F. Neurosurgery of the peripheral nervous system: cubital tunnel syndrome. Surg Neurol. 1998;50(1):83–5. https://doi.org/10.1016/s0090-3019(97)00231-0.
4. Bi AS, Qiu CS, Dellon AL, Rettig ME. A history of anatomical eponyms of the ulnar nerve. J Hand Surg Am. 2022;47(12):1211–7. https://doi.org/10.1016/j.jhsa.2022.09.013.
5. Brown JM, Mokhtee D, Evangelista MS, Mackinnon SE. Scratch collapse test localizes Osborne's band as the point of maximal nerve compression in cubital tunnel syndrome. Hand (NY). 2010;5(2):141–7. https://doi.org/10.1007/s11552-009-9225-4.
6. Davidge KM, Gontre G, Tang D, et al. The "hierarchical" scratch collapse test for identifying multilevel ulnar nerve compression. Hand (NY). 2015;10(3):388–95. https://doi.org/10.1007/s11552-014-9721-z.
7. Mezian K, Jačisko J, Kaiser R, et al. Ulnar neuropathy at the elbow: from ultrasound scanning to treatment. Front Neurol. 2021;12:661441. https://doi.org/10.3389/fneur.2021.661441.

8. Staples JR, Calfee R. Cubital tunnel syndrome: current concepts. J Am Acad Orthop Surg. 2017;25(10):e215–24. https://doi.org/10.5435/JAAOS-D-15-00261.
9. Svernlöv B, Larsson M, Rehn K, Adolfsson L. Conservative treatment of the cubital tunnel syndrome. J Hand Surg Eur. 2009;34(2):201–7. https://doi.org/10.1177/1753193408098480.
10. Biggs M, Curtis JA. Randomized, prospective study comparing ulnar neurolysis in situ with submuscular transposition. Neurosurgery. 2006;58(2):296–304.; discussion 296–304. https://doi.org/10.1227/01.NEU.0000194847.04143.A1.
11. Brauer CA, Graham B. The surgical treatment of cubital tunnel syndrome: a decision analysis. J Hand Surg Eur. 2007;32(6):654–62. https://doi.org/10.1016/J.JHSE.2007.07.001.
12. Mirza A, Reinhart MK, Bove J, Litwa J. Scope-assisted release of the cubital tunnel. J Hand Surg Am. 2011;36(1):147–51. https://doi.org/10.1016/j.jhsa.2010.10.016.
13. Koehler SM, Lovy AJ, Guerra SM, Chawla H, Hausman MR. Minimally invasive in situ cubital tunnel decompression. Tech Hand Up Extrem Surg. 2016;20(1):42–7. https://doi.org/10.1097/BTH.0000000000000113.
14. Karthik K, Nanda R, Storey S, Stothard J. Severe ulnar nerve entrapment at the elbow: functional outcome after minimally invasive in situ decompression. J Hand Surg Eur. 2012;37(2):115–22. https://doi.org/10.1177/1753193411416426.
15. Ochi K, Horiuchi Y, Nakamura T, Sato K, Arino H, Koyanagi T. Ulnar nerve strain at the elbow in patients with cubital tunnel syndrome: effect of simple decompression. J Hand Surg Eur. 2013;38(5):474–80. https://doi.org/10.1177/1753193412465234.
16. Poujade T, Hanouz N, Lecoq B, Hulet C, Collon S. Ultrasound-guided surgical treatment for ulnar nerve entrapment: a cadaver study. Chir Main. 2014;33(4):256–62. https://doi.org/10.1016/j.main.2014.05.006.
17. Guo D, Kliot M, McCool L, Senk A, Tonkin B, Guo D. Percutaneous cubital tunnel release with a dissection thread: a cadaveric study. J Hand Surg Eur. 2019;44(9):920–4. https://doi.org/10.1177/1753193419856591.
18. Mansour J, Ghanimeh J, Ghersi A, et al. Percutaneous ultrasound-guided ulnar nerve release technique compared to open technique: a cadaveric study. SICOT J. 2022;8:40. https://doi.org/10.1051/sicotj/2022041.
19. Dützmann S, Martin KD, Sobottka S, et al. Open vs retractor-endoscopic in situ decompression of the ulnar nerve in cubital tunnel syndrome: a retrospective cohort study. Neurosurgery. 2013;72(4):605–16.; discussion 614–616. https://doi.org/10.1227/NEU.0b013e3182846dbd.
20. Watts AC, Bain GI. Patient-rated outcome of ulnar nerve decompression: a comparison of endoscopic and open in situ decompression. J Hand Surg Am. 2009;34(8):1492–8. https://doi.org/10.1016/j.jhsa.2009.05.014.
21. Flores LP. Endoscopically assisted release of the ulnar nerve for cubital tunnel syndrome. Acta Neurochir. 2010;152(4):619–25. https://doi.org/10.1007/s00701-009-0578-9.

14 Epitrochleitis: Ultrasound-Guided Release

Olivier Mares and Vincent Martinel

14.1 Introduction

Medial epicondylitis (ME), also known as golfer's elbow, is a painful condition that affects the medial common flexor tendon at its insertion at the medial epicondyle [1]. Nowadays, the prevailing opinion is that ME is a degenerative process, as the histology shows a tendinosis [2].

Its main clinical feature is pain on the medial side of the elbow, during the flexion against resistance of the wrist and the formation of the fist. Conservative treatment is our first option with 90% success, leaving about 10% of refractory cases for surgery [3]. It is necessary to rule out the presence of an associated lacertus syndrome, performing a scratch collapse test.

Operative procedures for ME may be broadly grouped into two main categories: open or under ultrasound (US).

A new treatment system has been developed with US guidance for releasing the fascia of the flexor muscles at the medial epicondyle. This minimally invasive procedure using the Kemis® device (Newclip®) was originally designed for carpal ligament release [4].

This technique uses ultrasound imaging to guide the surgeon, allowing for precise localization of the affected area and targeted delivery treatment. It is a minimally invasive procedure that can be done on an outpatient basis, reducing the risk of complications associated with surgery such as bleeding or infection, allowing for a quicker recovery time, with an excellent cost efficiency ratio, compared to open surgery, obtaining favorable results in more than 90% of cases.

A preoperative examination is achieved to confirm the diagnosis.

14.2 Personal Technique

14.2.1 Indications

Patients with medial epicondylitis who have previously undergone conservative treatment for at least 6 months. This included oral NSAIDs, injection of hydrocortisone, platelet-rich plasma (PRP), or shockwave therapy.

14.2.2 Setup

We use a US high-frequency linear probe (GE) in B mode with a musculoskeletal preset at 13 MHz. A previous US examination is performed before sterile preparation of the arm. We start the procedure by first spotting the structures at risk: the

O. Mares (✉)
Department of Traumatology and Orthopedic Surgery, University Hospital Nîmes, Nimes, France

V. Martinel
Clinique de l'ormeau, Tarbes, France

O. Marès et al. (eds.), *Ultrasound-Guided Limb Surgery*,
https://doi.org/10.1007/978-3-031-88679-9_14

medial collateral ligament of the humero-ulnar joint and the ulnar nerve.

A sterile US transducer cover and gel are used to ensure sterility of the US probe throughout the entire procedure.

The patient is placed in the supine position, the affected arm on a hand table, elbow at 90° of flexion (Fig. 14.1). The medial aspect of the elbow is then prepared and sterile drapes are used in the usual fashion. Anesthesia is realized according to the protocol of wide awake local anesthesia no tourniquet (WALANT), with lidocaine plus epinephrine.

Then the flexor tendon fascia is identified in the coronal and frontal plane at a mean distance of 2 cm proximal to the medial epicondyle. The patient is asked to make active flexion of the wrist to visualize the medial collateral ligament insertion (Figs. 14.2a and 14.2b).

We identified the proximal zone of the section that must be far away from the ulnar nerve. The section is done from the ulnar crest in the direction of the biceps groove.

In a coronal view, a needle is passed beneath the fascia from the medial to the lateral side to ensure the best entry point for the device to release the fascia, without damaging any structure.

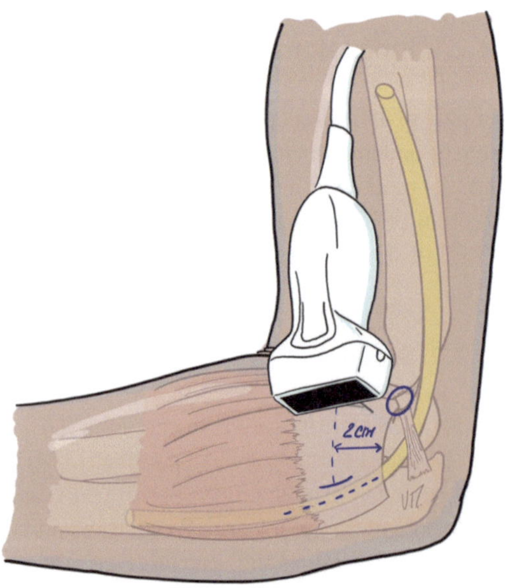

Fig. 14.1 Cutaneous landmark on the medial aspect

The skin is open on 0.5 cm and then smooth forceps are passed under the medial fascia on the deep part of the tendon (Figs. 14.3a and 14.3b).

The Kemis device is then inserted and is under full US guidance during all the procedure.

The section starts from the medial to the lateral side, the aponeurosis is cut, and the tendon is released. The aim is to release the fascia to obtain a large lengthening of the medial muscle mass of the epicondyle. Smooth forceps are passed to be sure to have completely released the tendon on a transverse view.

The skin is not closed, applying just a bulky dressing for 24 h. The wound healing is obtained in 2/3 days (Picture 14.1).

14.2.3 Pearls and Pitfalls

To prevent incomplete medial fascia release, minimally invasive surgical knives are more effective than needle techniques, which merely scratch the fascia. Complete sectioning of the fascia is ensured after the knife's passage. Ensuring the entry point and the knife's trajectory with a needle is necessary and must be time-consuming. Once positioned correctly, the knife entraps the fascia, and a transverse view of the Kemis ensures the good position before starting to cut the fascia in an "in-plane" view.

To avoid neurovascular damage, several precautions are essential. Firstly, marking the ulnar nerve direction on the skin is critical. Some patients experienced a kind of skin depression at the section level due to the lengthening of the fascia. This depression is a transitory effect and will disappear with the healing of the tendon in 2/3 months.

The patient is asked to use his arms immediately after the procedure. We advocate no specific immobilization. Physiotherapy is initiated a few days after surgery. Heavy activities are encouraged after 8 weeks. Postoperative analgesia is prescribed with level one classic painkillers with nonsteroidal anti-inflammatory drugs (NSAIDs) for 1 week.

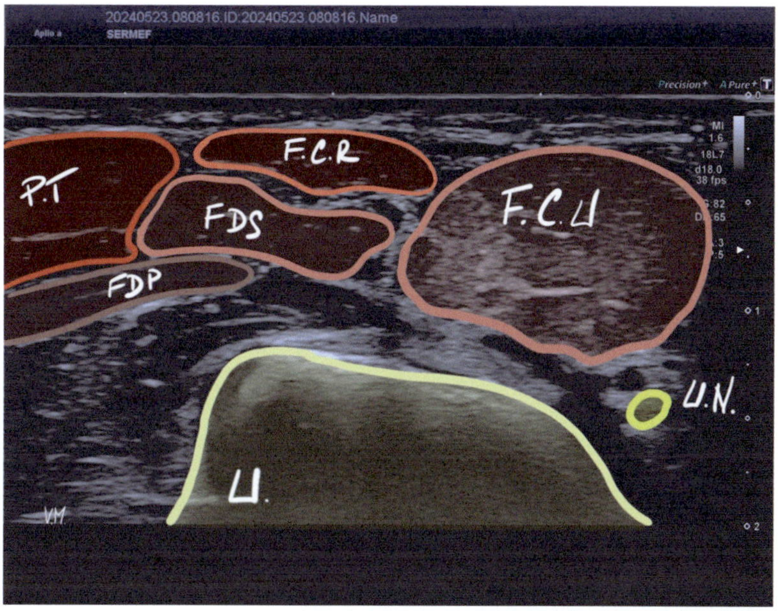

Fig. 14.2a Transverse view medial fascia, flexor muscles, ligament. *FCR* flexor carpi radialis, *FCU* flexor carpi ulnaris, *FDP* flexor digital profundus, *FDS* flexor digital superficialis, *PT* pronator teres, *U* ulnar bone, *UN* ulnar nerve

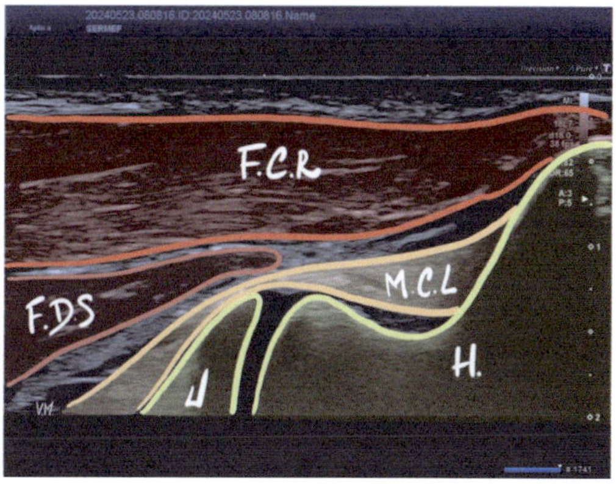

Fig. 14.2b Ultrasound longitudinal view of the medial fascia. *FCR* flexor carpi radialis, *FDS* flexor digital superficialis, *H* humeral bone, *MCL* medial collateral ligament

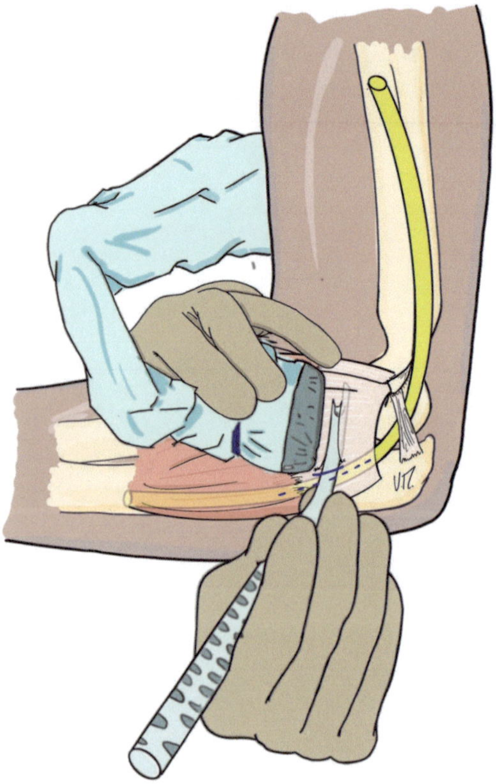

Fig. 14.3a Schematic view of the section

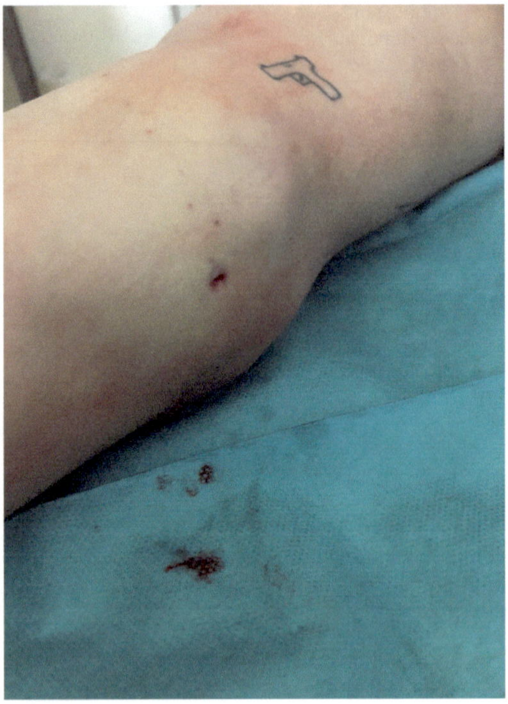

Picture 14.1 size of the wound

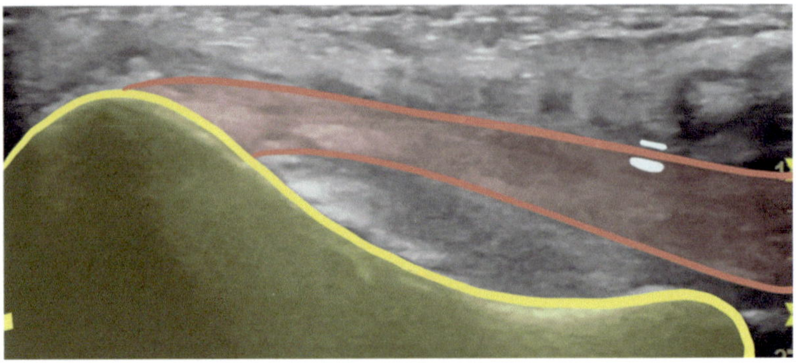

Fig. 14.3b Ultrasound view: section of the medial fascia: transverse view with the miniKemis (Newclip Technics) knife during section at distance of the medial ligament of the humero-ulnar articulation and ulnar nerve

Take-Home Messages

Indication

Patient with surgery indications for epitochleitis resistant to medical treatment

Contraindication

Patients with ulnar nerve compression, medial elbow instability, and intra-articular pathology on the medial aspect of the elbow

Surgical technique

(a) WALANT anesthesia is done with 20/30 CC
(b) The patient is placed in the supine position, the affected arm on a hand table, elbow at 90° of flexion
(c) The proximal zone of the section that must be far away from the ulnar nerve
(d) Ultrasound is used to assess the position of the safe zone
(e) The entry point is found with a needle
(f) Open the skin with a knife with a 0.5 cm incision
(g) The cutting device is passed under the fascia under ultrasound control. The procedure is done until the ligament is cut.
(h) Control the release with a Halstead forceps.

Postoperative care

(i) Dressing for 48 h is essential to avoid hematoma.
(j) Free use of the hand is authorized immediately.

Conclusion

Ultrasound release of the common flexor tendon is feasible and reproducible with this mini-invasive technique. The recovery allows a quick return to daily activities.

The full recovery of the flexor strength is obtained in the mean of 6 months.

Approximately 8% of our patients, particularly those with significant preoperative pain levels, may experience persistent pain or motion limitations. However, these issues generally diminish by the 3-month mark—a point we communicate clearly to patients preoperatively to align their expectations. On rare occasions, a postoperative corticosteroid injection may be necessary, which typically leads to symptom resolution.

Bibliography

1. Leach RE, Miller JK. Lateral and medial epicondylitis of the elbow. Clin Sports Med. 1987;6(2):259–72.
2. Kraushaar BS, Nirschl RP. Tendinosis of the elbow (tennis elbow). Clinical features and findings of histological, immunohistochemical, and electron microscopy studies. J Bone Joint Surg Am. 1999;81(2):259–78.
3. Lowdon H, Chong HH, Dhingra M, Gomaa AR, Teece L, Booth S, Watts AC, Singh HP. Comparison of interventions for lateral elbow tendinopathy: a systematic review and network meta-analysis for patient-rated tennis elbow evaluation pain outcome. J Hand Surg Am. 2024;S0363-5023(24):00104–7.
4. Apard T, Candelier G. Surgical ultrasound-guided carpal tunnel release. Hand Surg Rehabil. 2017;36(5):333–7.

Part V

Forearm

15 Lacertus Syndrome Antegrade Ultrasound-Guided Technique

Olivier Marès

15.1 Introduction

Lacertus syndrome, when diagnosed, requires appropriate care [1]. The first therapeutic option is medical. It combines an ultrasound-guided injection of cortisone derivative under the lacertus near the median nerve, with manual fasciatherapy work. When this option is insufficient and does not provide relief, it is then necessary to release this aponeurotic expansion, which generates this dynamic compression [2].

We describe a proximal to distal release technique, performed under ultrasound-guided control and WALANT-type local anesthesia.

15.2 Personal Technique

15.2.1 Anesthesia

The injection begins 1 cm above the elbow crease; we then perform four injection points separated by 2 cm from proximal to distal with 4 cc each time.

3 cc are then injected under the fascia in order to obtain complete painlessness when performing the procedure.

The waiting time before starting is less than 5 min because the analgesic block is quick. This is a percutaneous surgery and there is no need to wait for the vascular effect. The use of adrenaline makes it possible to avoid stopping patients' anticoagulants and increase the analgesic block with an average duration of 8–10 h.

15.2.2 Patient Installation

The patient is in a supine position with his arm on a hand table without a tourniquet.

15.2.3 Skin Identification

The incision point is 1 cm upstream of the elbow crease (Fig. 15.1). The longitudinal line of work is identified using ultrasound identification. The objective is to be at a distance from both the great vessels of the elbow crease and the median nerve. The incision is more medial or ulnar than the open incision.

You must take the time to take care of this identification—it is one of the keys to the success of this surgery.

Supplementary Information The online version contains supplementary material available at https://doi.org/10.1007/978-3-031-88679-9_15.

O. Marès (✉)
Department of Traumatology and Orthopedic Surgery, University Hospital Nîmes, Nîmes, France

O. Marès et al. (eds.), *Ultrasound-Guided Limb Surgery*,
https://doi.org/10.1007/978-3-031-88679-9_15

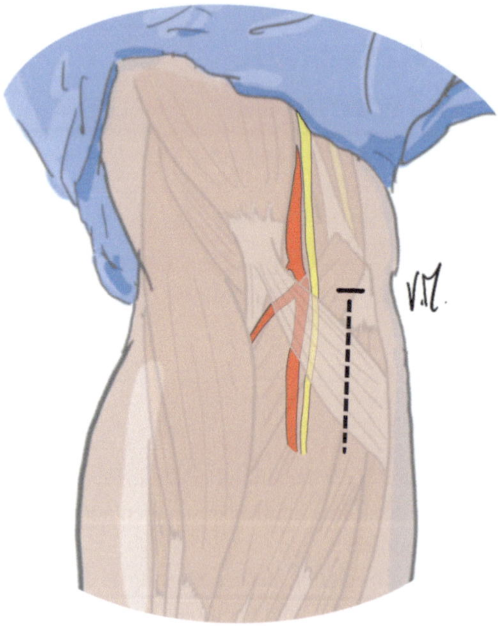

Fig. 15.1 Skin identification of the incision and the different anatomical structures. (Artwork by Vincent Martinel, reproduced with permission)

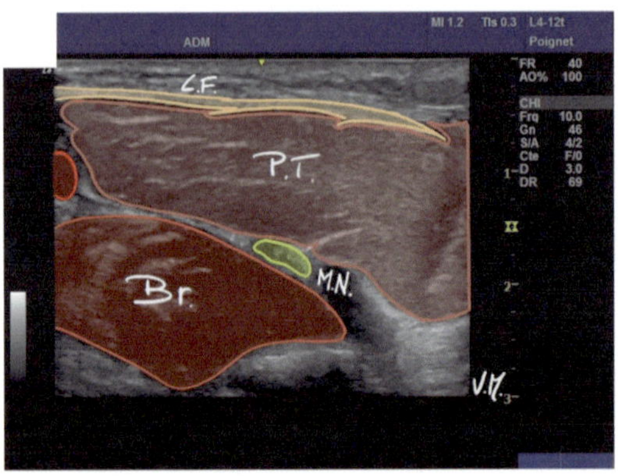

Fig. 15.2a Cross section: the median nerve is under the pronator teres

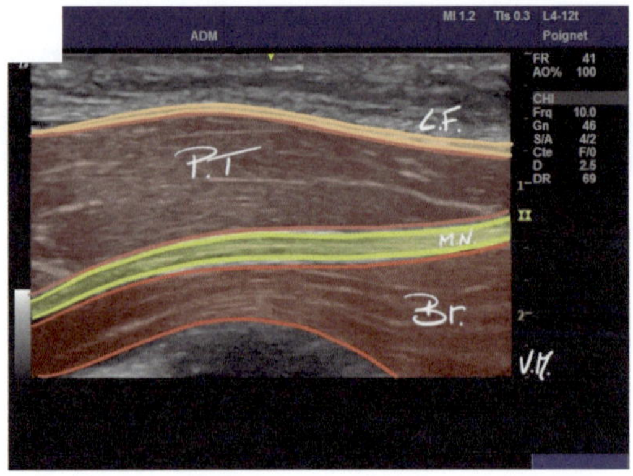

Fig. 15.2b Longitudinal view: the median nerve is at a distance from the lacertus, which is superficial to the pronator teres. In yellow the median nerve; *PT* pronator teres, *BR* brachioradialis. (Artwork by Vincent Martinel, reproduced with permission)

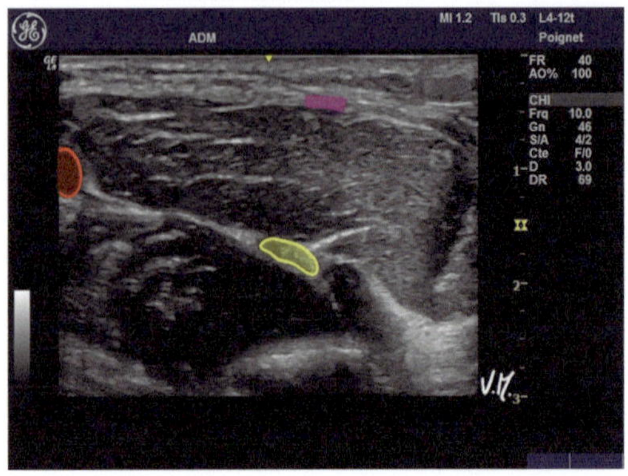

Fig. 15.3 Cross section: the lower blade of the knife is visualized in purple on the section. In yellow the median nerve; *PT* pronator teres, *BR* brachioradialis. (Artwork by Vincent Martinel, reproduced with permission)

15.2.4 Surgical Procedure

Repair of the different structures is carried out with transverse and longitudinal ultrasound control (Figs. 15.2a and 15.2b). A skin speckle is made with a 15-blade scalpel. Then a Halstead forceps is introduced and positioned under the lacertus. Its positioning is checked on a longitudinal and transverse section.

A specific knife is then introduced through the incision. The positioning of the knife is sought on a cross section (Fig. 15.3). The lower part of the knife should be under the aponeurosis away from the vessels, which are in a lateral position, and the median nerve, which is under the pronator teres muscle.

Then the section is carried out on a longitudinal control until complete release is obtained (Fig. 15.4).

Intraoperative testing shows the disappearance of the scratch collapse test and the recovery of force on the flexor pollicis longus and the flexor digitorum profundus.

15.2.5 Closure

A hydrocellular dressing is positioned and a pressure bandage is maintained for 24 h (Fig. 15.5).

Then, the patient performs his own care by cleaning with mild soap and applying a simple dressing. Resumption of daily activities is carried out on the same day of the operation. The resumption of strength activities, particularly those with vibrations, is resumed from the third week.

Patients regain strength from the day of the procedure, but relief of their symptoms is optimal between 6 and 8 weeks.

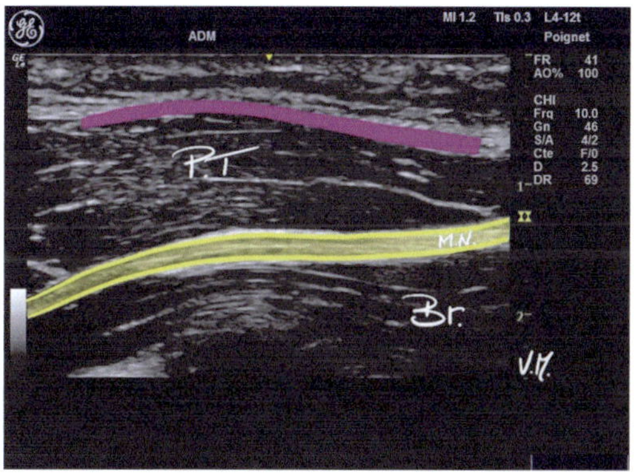

Fig. 15.4 Longitudinal section: in purple the section area of the lacertus. In yellow the median nerve; *PT* pronator teres, *BR* brachioradialis. (Artwork by Vincent Martinel, reproduced with permission)

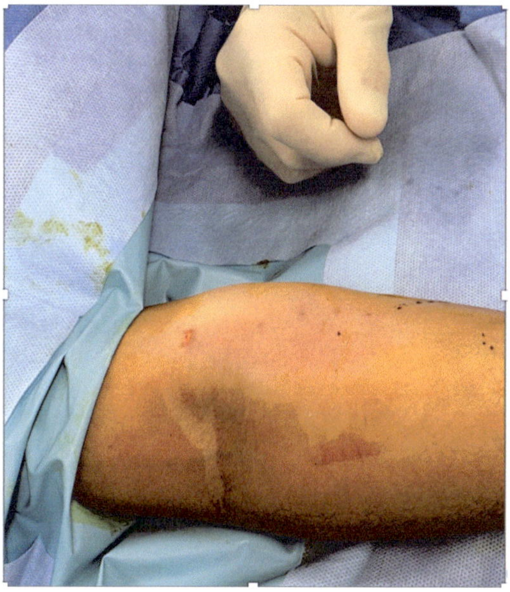

Fig. 15.5 Scar

15.3 Tips and Tricks

Positioning of the incision to avoid complications and incomplete releases.

The use of WALANT reduces the risk of hematoma and reduces postoperative pain compared to simple local anesthesia.

This technique is not recommended in patients with a high BMI, because the thickness of the subcutaneous fatty tissue can hinder the performance of the procedure.

You should not incise flush with the biceps, nor have a path from medial to lateral, because there is a risk of damaging the superficial veins of the elbow crease.

A pressure dressing is applied systematically.

15.4 Complications

If the different steps are followed correctly, the only risk is a hematoma of the forearm, which is exceptionally compressive (Fig. 15.6). Most of the time, it resolves in 3/4 weeks with local care.

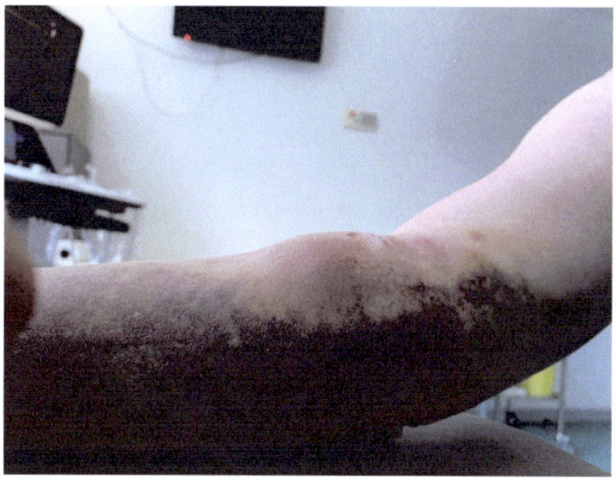

Fig. 15.6 Postoperative hematoma

15.5 Conclusion

Ultrasound release of the lacertus is feasible and reproducible with this mini-invasive technique. The recovery allows a return to sport in 3 weeks and a return to performance in 6 weeks. The only risk is a hematoma or if the section is done too close to the biceps a neuroma of a superficial branch.

Take-Home Messages

Indication

Patient with surgery indications for lacertus.

After the failure of the medical treatment: strapping, injection.

Contraindication

Patients with vascular deformity such as superficial artery or cyst.

Surgical Technique

WALANT anesthesia 20/30 CC; from the proximal of the elbow joint crease in the axis of the median nerve on a length of 10 cm.

The aim is to find the safe zone between the medial side of the biceps and the vessels and the deep structure of the median nerve.

Find the best entry point with a 25-gauge needle 1 cm proximal to the flexion crease and 2 cm medial of the medial border of the biceps tendon. On a transverse view, the needle should be under the lacertus band, 2 cm up from the median nerve, and 1.5 cm away from the vessels.

Open the skin with a knife to 1 cm.

Pass a Halstead forceps under the skin to feel the lacertus. The probe assesses the good position of the forceps as in C.

The Halstead should be passed up and down the lacertus to free the small veins.

The knife is inserted on a transverse view to assess the good position.

The section is done on an in-plane view to control the full release of the band.

Control the release with a Halstead forceps.

Postoperative care

Pressure dressing for 48 h is essential to avoid hematoma.

Free use of the hand is authorized immediately.

References

1. Hagert E, Jedeskog U, Hagert CG, Marín FT. Lacertus syndrome: a ten year analysis of two hundred and seventy five minimally invasive surgical decompressions of median nerve entrapment at the elbow. Int Orthop. 2023;47(4):1005–11. https://doi.org/10.1007/s00264-023-05709-w. Epub 2023 Feb 9
2. Apard T, Martinel V, Batby G, Draznieks G, Descamps J. Lacertus syndrome: recent advances. Hand Surg Rehabil. 2024;7:101738.

16 Percutaneous Ultrasound-Guided Release of the Lacertus Fibrosus

Thomas Apard

16.1 Introduction

The compression of the median nerve around the elbow is less frequent than at the carpal tunnel [1, 2]. Nevertheless, this underestimated condition has long since been recognized as the pronator syndrome [2–4]. It is due to the dynamic compression of the median nerve as it courses through the pronator teres [5, 6]. Merging with the perimuscular fascia of the pronator teres, as well as superficially surrounding the muscle, the lacertus fibrosus (LF) of the biceps brachii contributes to this compression [7, 8].

Because electromyographic and imaging studies of the median nerve frequently remain normal or nonspecific [4–6, 9], the diagnosis of the syndrome relies on the specific clinical triad of Hagert including weakness of muscles innervated by the median nerve, pain at compression of the cubital fossa of the elbow, and positive scratch collapse test [4, 5, 10].

Decompression can be considered if symptoms persist after 3–6 months of conservative management [5, 6]. Decompressive surgeries have been refined over time from deep extensive release of the median nerve [2, 11] to more simple superficial releases of the LF. These are still performed in an operating room under general or locoregional anesthesia, using a tourniquet to control bleeding [12, 13]. In comparison, wide-awake local anesthesia no tourniquet (WALANT) has been developed and now allows the execution of a variety of surgeries [20], including the release of the LF [4], with optimal comfort plus excellent control of bleeding.

The ultrasound-guided release of the carpal tunnel is now validated [15, 16]. As the superficial fascia of the pronator teres muscle is visible with high-resolution transducers [17], with no major nerve or vessel crossing the area of intervention [7, 8], a similar technique may be considered for pronator syndrome.

16.2 Personal Technique (Video 1)

Surgery indication includes definite pronator syndrome with significant impairment of usual activities, visual analog scale (VAS) pain score equal to or greater than 3 out of 10, and failure of conservative management. The diagnosis is confirmed by the positivity of all three signs of Hagert's triad. In particular, the strength of the flexor pollicis longus and flexor digitorum profundus of the second finger must be unequivo-

Supplementary Information The online version contains supplementary material available at https://doi.org/10.1007/978-3-031-88679-9_16.

T. Apard (✉)
Centre Echochirurgie de la Main, Versailles, France

O. Marès et al. (eds.), *Ultrasound-Guided Limb Surgery*,
https://doi.org/10.1007/978-3-031-88679-9_16

cally reduced. Exclusion criteria are as follows: concurrent carpal tunnel surgery, intrinsic tumor or focal lesion with direct compression of the median nerve, systemic nerve disease, and lidocaine allergy.

First, with no preoperative fasting, patients are set up in an interventional ultrasound room. Using ultrasound, the path of the brachial artery is traced on the skin. Then, the transducer is slightly moved medially to visualize the brachial artery in the top left corner of the image, plus the median nerve deep to the belly of the pronator teres. The proximal edge of the muscle is marked as the most proximal boundary of the procedure. Then, avoiding major subcutaneous veins, the cutaneous entry point is marked distally enough to allow the release of the fascia of the pronator teres over a distance of 4–5 cm (Fig. 16.1a, b).

Second, local anesthesia is performed 30 min preoperatively with 30–40 ml of WALANT solution, totaling a maximum injected dose of 200 mg of lidocaine. In our institution, the solution is prepared in 12 ml syringes by a mixture of 5 ml of 1% lidocaine—10 mg/ml—plus epinephrine 5 μg/ml with 5 ml of normal saline, and 1 ml sodium bicarbonate 8.4%. It is injected in the subcutaneous tissue of the cubital fossa under ultrasound guidance to avoid any anesthesia-induced paralysis of the median nerve. The anesthetic extends from the elbow crease to 5 cm distally and covered the perimuscular fascia of the pronator teres medial to the main tendon of the biceps brachii (Fig. 16.2).

Muscle weakness is then retested to confirm the diagnosis and rule out anesthesia-induced pain block as a cause of returned muscle strength (Fig. 16.3).

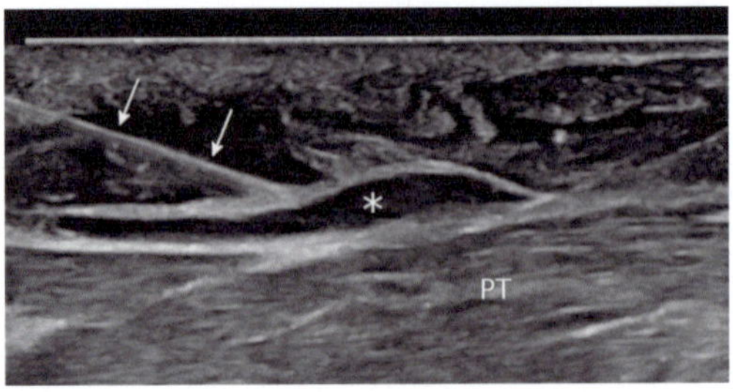

Fig. 16.2 Local anesthesia. *Arrows:* needle, asterisk: diffusion of the WALANT solution superficial to the perimuscular fascia of the pronator teres; *PT* pronator teres muscle

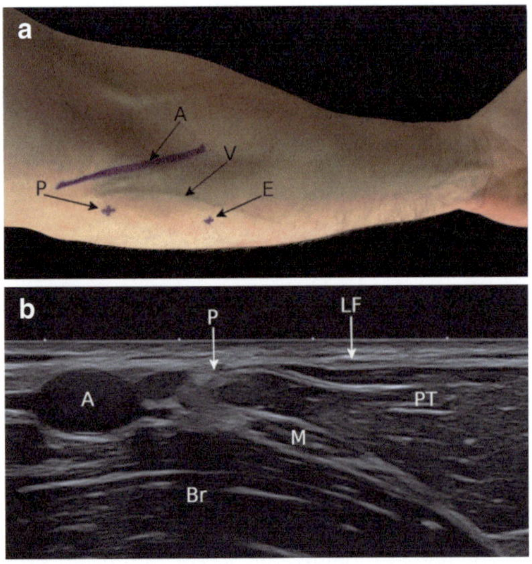

Fig. 16.1 Preprocedural planning. (**a**) Preprocedural cutaneous marking. (**b**) Preprocedural ultrasound view. *A* figurative path of the brachial artery, *M* median nerve, *P* proximal edge of the pronator teres, *E* cutaneous entry point, *V* superficial vein, *LF* lacertus fibrosus, *PT* pronator teres muscle, *Br* brachialis muscle

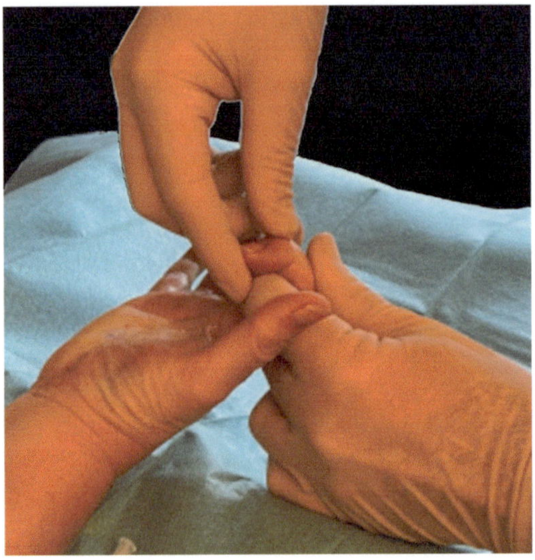

Fig. 16.3 Testing for confirmation of muscle weakness. Note that the test is performed with flexion of the two interphalangeal joints

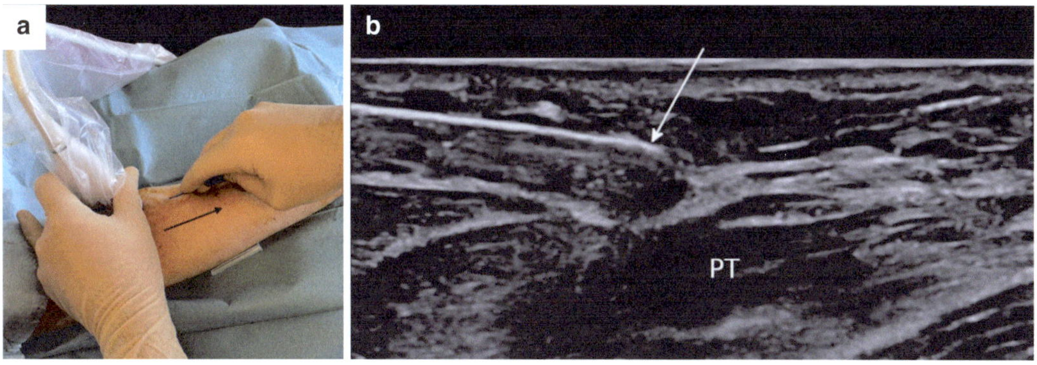

Fig. 16.4 Ongoing retrograde release of the lacertus fibrosus. (**a**) Positioning of both retrograde knife and ultrasound probe. (**b**) In-plane ultrasound view. *Arrow:* hook of the retrograde knife; *PT* pronator teres muscle

Third, the release of the LF is performed under "in-plane" ultrasound guidance (Video 1) with an ECTRA II retrograde hook knife (Smith and Nephew®, France). After a millimetric skin incision, the hook is proximally advanced superficial to the pronator teres until it reaches the predefined proximal edge of the muscle. At this point, the knife is rotated to hook this edge and the LF is cut retrogradely under constant monitoring of both the brachial artery and the median nerve (Fig. 16.4).

Finally, a circular soft dressing is applied for 24 h. Mobilization is encouraged the day after the procedure and time off work is limited to a few days. Follow-up is conducted with visits at postoperative weeks 1 and 4, including strength testing, VAS scoring, and assessment for complications.

16.3 Results

Since 2016, we operated more than 700 lacertus syndromes percutaneously under ultrasound.

No perioperative complication occurred, including injury to any notable structure. Twelve percent of patients presented a hematoma (from 3 to 7 cm long), which completely resorbed by week 4 except for three patients (0.4%) who had been reoperated with open surgery to drain it.

No major delayed complication occurred. The cutaneous incisions easily healed with no inadvertent scar tissue (no keloid as we used to observe with vertical incision of the anterior forearm). No infection occurred.

WALANT allowed the completion of all procedures. Neither additional injection of numbing solution nor systemic analgesic medication was required. No complication due to either lidocaine or epinephrine occurred.

16.4 Discussion

By providing significant advantages over traditional techniques, the concurrent use of ultrasound guidance and WALANT anesthesia allows the microinvasive release of the LF superficial to the belly of the pronator teres. At least in the short term, the technique yields high success rates appearing similar to those reported with more invasive surgical interventions [4, 12, 13].

With real-time monitoring of major nerves and vessels, including uncommon variations [18, 19], ultrasound guidance secures the procedure. The millimetric incision should limit the formation of scar tissue [20] and allow easier recovery [21].

As WALANT preserves both the contractility of muscles and normal consciousness of the patient [4, 14], the operator can test the recovery of strength perioperatively to ensure that proper release is achieved [4]. With a dose of lidocaine being far below the maximum recommended dose of 500 mg [22], the anesthesia can be performed outside the operating room by nonanesthesiologist physicians. With bleeding being controlled by the vasoconstriction induced by epinephrine, no uncomfortable tourniquet is needed [23].

16.5 Conclusion

Combined with WALANT anesthesia, the micro-invasive ultrasound-guided release of the LF superficial to the belly of the pronator teres could be a valuable treatment of lacertus syndrome.

Take-Home Messages

Indication

Proximal median nerve compression syndrome (lacertus syndrome) with conservative treatment failure

Contraindication

Concurrent carpal tunnel surgery

Intrinsic tumor of focal lesion with direct compression of the median nerve

Systemic nerve disease

Lidocaine allergy

Surgical Technique

(a) US examination with braquial artery pathway and proximal edge of pronator teres muscle marked in the skin
(b) Local anesthesia with 30–40 ml of WALANT solution. Maximum injected dose of 200 mg of lidocaine
(c) “In-plane” release of the LF
(d) Hook knife superficial to the pronator teres fascia
(e) 3 mm skin incision with a 15-blade parallel
(f) Subcutaneous dissection with a Halsted forceps. Pierce the fascia. Control the position of the instrument on a transverse and longitudinal view
(g) Knife introduction. Verify on transverse and longitudinal view
(h) Gently push the knife distally (holding your probe horizontaly) to release the fascia as far as possible
(i) Check the complete freeing of the fascia using a Halsted forceps

Postoperative care

Circular soft dressing

Mobility in encourage 24 h after surgery

Bibliography

1. Latinovic R. Incidence of common compressive neuropathies in primary care. J Neurol Neurosurg Psychiatry. 2006;77:263–5. https://doi.org/10.1136/jnnp.2005.066696.
2. Hartz CR, Linscheid RL, Gramse RR, Daube JR. The pronator teres syndrome: compressive neuropathy of the median nerve. J Bone Joint Surg Am. 1981;63:885–90.
3. Seyffart H. Primary myoses in the m. pronator teres as cause of lesion of the n. medianus (the pronator syndrome). Acta Psychiatr Neurol Scand Suppl. 1951;74:251–4.
4. Hagert E. Clinical diagnosis and wide-awake surgical treatment of proximal median nerve entrapment at the elbow: a prospective study. Hand. 2013;8:41–6. https://doi.org/10.1007/s11552-012-9483-4.
5. Adler JA, Wolf JM. Proximal median nerve compression: pronator syndrome. J Hand Surg Am. 2020;45:1157–65. https://doi.org/10.1016/j.jhsa.2020.07.006.
6. Dang AC, Rodner CM. Unusual compression neuropathies of the forearm, part II: median nerve. J Hand Surg Am. 2009;34:1915–20. https://doi.org/10.1016/j.jhsa.2009.10.017.
7. Eames MH, Bain GI, Fogg QA, Van Riet RP. Distal biceps tendon anatomy: a cadaveric study. J Bone Joint Surg Am. 2007;89:1044–9. https://doi.org/10.2106/JBJS.D.02992.
8. Snoeck O, Lefèvre P, Sprio E, et al. The lacertus fibrosus of the biceps brachii muscle: an anatomical study. Surg Radiol Anat. 2014;36:713–9. https://doi.org/10.1007/s00276-013-1254-6.
9. El-Haj M, Ding W, Sharma K, Novak C, Mackinnon SE, Patterson JM. Median nerve compression in the forearm: a clinical diagnosis. Hand (NY). 2021;16:586–91. https://doi.org/10.1177/1558944719874137.
10. Jiménez I, Delgado PJ. The scratch collapse test in the diagnosis of compression of the median nerve in the proximal forearm. J Hand Surg Eur. 2017;42:937–40. https://doi.org/10.1177/1753193417726214.
11. Nigst H, Dick W. Syndromes of compression of the median nerve in the proximal forearm (pronator teres syndrome; anterior interosseous nerve syndrome).

Arch Orthop Trauma Surg. 1979;93:307–12. https://doi.org/10.1007/BF00450231.
12. Zancolli ER, Zancolli EPIV, Perrotto CJ. New mini-invasive decompression for pronator teres syndrome. J Hand Surg Am. 2012;37:1706–10. https://doi.org/10.1016/j.jhsa.2012.05.033.
13. Vergara-Amador E, Castillo-Pérez S, Tovar-Cuellar W. Endoscopic release of the median nerve in the proximal third of the forearm. A new approach. Rev Esp Cir Ortop Traumatol (Eng Ed). 2019;63:439–46. https://doi.org/10.1016/j.recot.2019.05.001.
14. Kurtzman JS, Etcheson JI, Koehler SM. Wide-awake local anesthesia with no tourniquet: an updated review. Plast Recon Surg Glob Open. 2021;9:e3507. https://doi.org/10.1097/GOX.0000000000003507.
15. Nakamichi K, Tachibana S. Ultrasonographically assisted carpal tunnel release. J Hand Surg Am. 1997;22:853–62. https://doi.org/10.1016/s0363-5023(97)80081-0.
16. Apard T, Candelier G. Surgical ultrasound-guided carpal tunnel release. Hand Surg Rehabil. 2017;36:333–7. https://doi.org/10.1016/j.hansur.2017.05.005.
17. Konschake M, Stofferin H, Moriggl B. Ultrasound visualization of an underestimated structure: the bicipital aponeurosis. Surg Radiol Anat. 2017;39:1317–22. https://doi.org/10.1007/s00276-017-1885-0.
18. Chakravarthi KK, Siddaraju KS, Nelluri Venumadhav AS, Kumar N. Anatomical variations of brachial artery—its morphology, embryogenesis and clinical implications. J Clin Diag Res. 2014;8:AC17–20. https://doi.org/10.7860/JCDR/2014/10418.5308.
19. Eid N, Ito Y, Shibata MA, Otsuki Y. Persistent median artery: cadaveric study and review of the literature. Clin Anat. 2011;24:627–33. https://doi.org/10.1002/ca.21127.
20. Tsai TM, Syed SA. A transverse skin incision approach for decompression of pronator teres syndrome. J Hand Surg Br. 1994;19:40–2. https://doi.org/10.1016/0266-7681(94)90047-7.
21. Rojo-Manaute JM, Capa-Grasa A, Chana-Rodriguez F, Perez-Mañanes R, Rodriguez-Maruri G, Sanz-Ruiz P, et al. Ultra-minimally invasive ultrasound-guided carpal tunnel release: a randomized clinical trial. J Ultrasound Med. 2016;35:1149–57. https://doi.org/10.7863/ultra.15.07001.
22. Rosenberg PH, Veering BT, Urmey WF. Maximum recommended doses of local anesthetics: a multifactorial concept. Reg Anesth Pain Med. 2004;29:564–75. https://doi.org/10.1016/j.rapm.2004.08.003.
23. Far-Riera AM, Pérez-Uribarri C, Jiménez MS, Serrano ME, González JR, Hernández IR. Prospective study on the application of a WALANT circuit. Rev Esp Cir Ortop Traumatol (Eng Ed). 2019;63:400–7. https://doi.org/10.1016/j.recot.2019.06.006.

17 Ultrasound-Guided Biceps Tenotomy

Sarah Pradel and Olivier Mares

17.1 Introduction

The biceps brachii primarily functions in flexion and supination of the elbow. The short head suspends the humerus and inserts via the conjoint tendon at the level of the coracoid process. Meanwhile, the long head of the biceps brachii inserts on the glenoid tubercle and stabilizes the humeral head, thus preventing its ascent under the acromion [1–4].

Long biceps tendinopathy is a prevalent condition, often resulting from subacromial impingement that leads to rotator cuff tears; the humeral head ascends and the tendon, representing the final brake to this ascent, is then overused. The long biceps tendon's long portion has a particular trajectory with a 90° zone that undergoes significant stresses [2]. The tendon hypertrophies with decreased sliding in the groove, exacerbating the pain; thus, the vicious cycle is closed [2, 3, 5].

Clinically, in most cases, anterior pain is found at the level of the bicipital groove, with nocturnal exacerbations and increased pain during the performance of clinical tests.

There are several conservative therapies available (rehabilitation, infiltration, adapted pain management, etc.) [6, 7], but when these prove ineffective, surgery becomes necessary. Tenotomy is indicated when medical treatment fails for rotator cuff tears in elderly individuals with a massive irreparable cuff tear without severe associated arthropathy or in cases of significant labral lesions [8, 9].

Numerous studies have highlighted similar functional outcomes between tenotomy associated with tenodesis or isolated tenotomy [10–13]. The latter improves functional results, increases mobility, and reduces pain, with an increased risk of proximal migration of the tenomuscular unit giving rise to the Popeye sign.

Long-head biceps tenotomy is usually performed arthroscopically in the operating room under general anesthesia or regional anesthesia with sedation [14]. Ultrasound-guided surgery makes it possible to manage chronic tendinopathies through tenotomy without arthroscopy and under local anesthesia, in the context of office-based surgery [15]. Ultrasound-guided biceps tenotomy was first described in 2005 in animals [16, 17].

17.2 Personal Technique

17.2.1 Indications

Long biceps tendinopathy is indicated in patients with anesthesia-related vulnerabilities who cannot undergo shoulder arthroplasty surgery and/or present with a massive irreparable rotator cuff tear.

S. Pradel · O. Mares (✉)
Department of Traumatology and Orthopedic Surgery, University Hospital Nîmes, Nîmes, France

O. Marès et al. (eds.), *Ultrasound-Guided Limb Surgery*,
https://doi.org/10.1007/978-3-031-88679-9_17

17.2.2 Contraindications

Ultrasound-guided biceps percutaneous tenotomy is contraindicated in young individuals, with or without reparable rotator cuff tear, or candidates for shoulder arthroplasty without medical condition contraindications.

17.2.3 Equipment

The equipment required to perform this technique is [18] shown in Fig. 17.1:

- An ultrasound machine with high-definition graphics (GE Logiq E ®)
- A high-frequency linear probe (> 12 Hz)
- Ultrasound gel and a sterile cover
- One (or two) 20 cc syringes with xylocaine +/− adrenaline
- A 21-gauge trocar
- A scalpel with a no.11 blade or a beaver

17.2.4 Operative Technique

Adjust the ultrasound machine settings according to the patient's echogenicity, adapting the depth, focus, and gain.

The first step involves positioning the upper limb in external rotation and supination (Fig. 17.2).

Next, perform ultrasound-guided localization of the tendon (Fig. 17.3) in the short and long axis. The procedure is performed under local anesthesia with 1% xylocaine +/− adrenaline. To better visualize the tendon within the groove, local anesthesia should be administered into the groove.

Before making the skin incision, locate the trajectory using a 21-gauge trocar (Figs. 17.4 and 17.5). The satisfactory trajectory involves positioning the trocar under the tendon.

Then, make the skin incision using a beaver, and advance the blade along the same trajectory

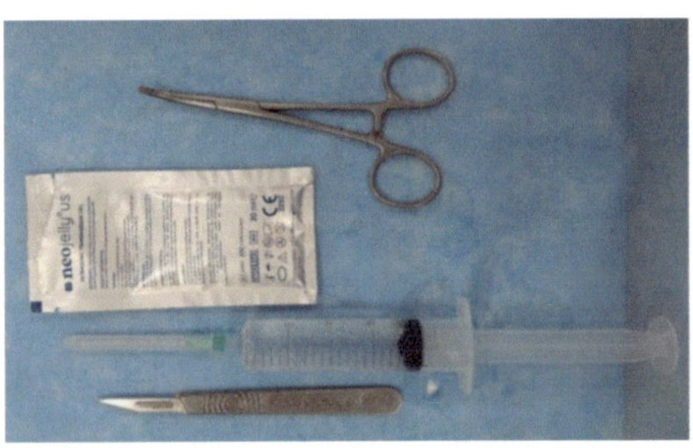

Fig. 17.1 Equipment required for ultrasound-guided tenotomy technique

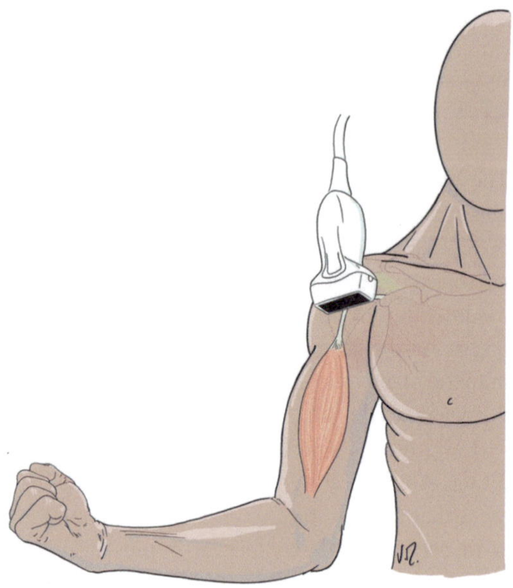

Fig. 17.2 Positing of the arm with the upper limb in supination. (Artwork by Vincent Martinel, reproduced with permission)

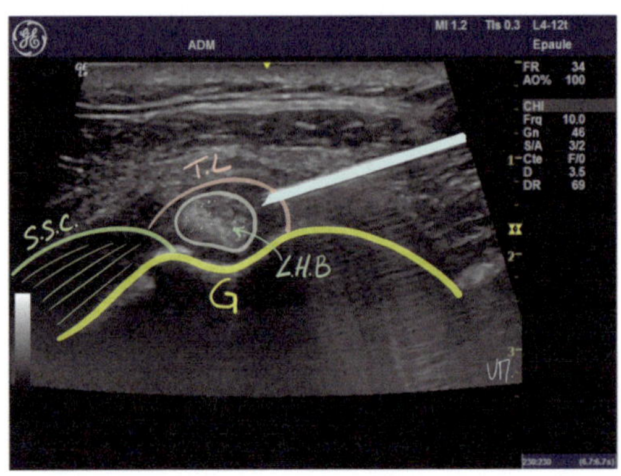

Fig. 17.3 Transverse view of the needle for the WALANT. (Artwork by Vincent Martinel, reproduced with permission)

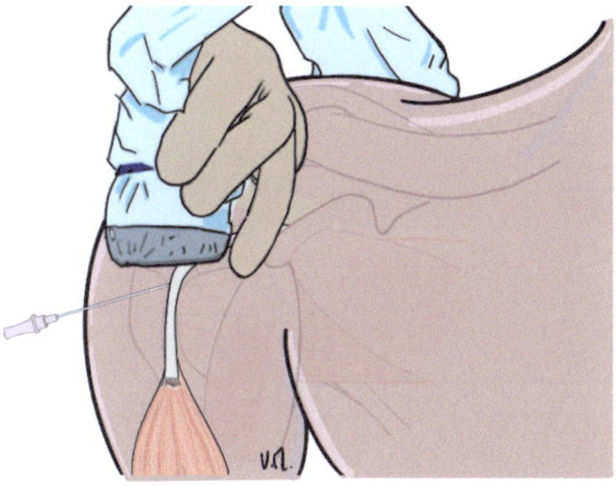

Fig. 17.4 Positing of the ultrasound probe and localization of the trajectory with the 21-gauge trocar. (Artwork by Vincent Martinel, reproduced with permission)

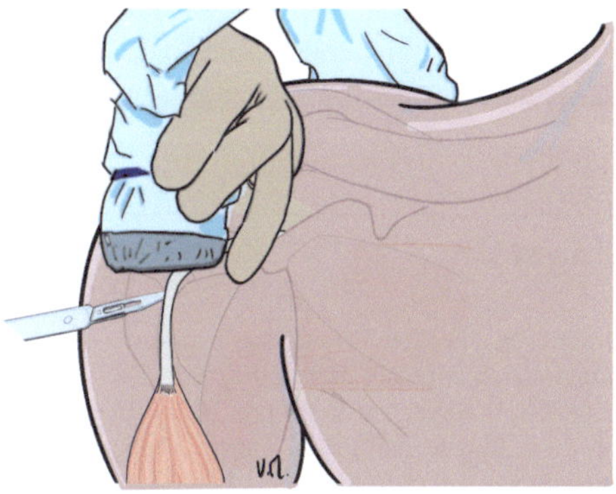

Fig. 17.5 Image of trajectory localization in-plane. (Artwork by Vincent Martinel, reproduced with permission)

until it contacts the posterior aspect of the tendon within the groove (Fig. 17.6). Insert the blade under the tendon and then perform a 90° rocking motion to bring the blade into contact with the tendon. Subsequently, perform posterior-to-anterior movements to section the tendon. A distinct crunching sound may be audible and perceptible. Maintain the limb in external rotation and supination to tension the tendon and facilitate the procedure.

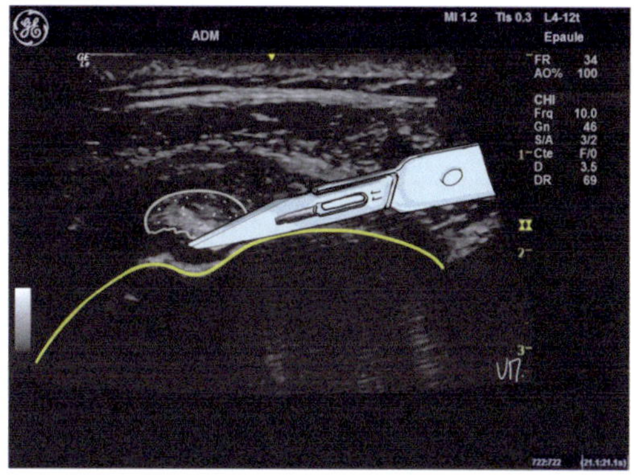

Fig. 17.6 An ultrasound image in-plane view of the scalpel blade positioning under the long biceps tendon at the biceps groove. (Artwork by Vincent Martinel, reproduced with permission)

17.3 Postoperative Care

At the end of the procedure, no suture is applied at the incision, and a simple dressing and no splint is advocated.

The patient may use their upper limb from the same day without any activity restrictions and can undergo rehabilitation sessions without restrictions. These sessions may include shoulder realignment/lowering physiotherapy and deltoid strengthening exercises.

17.4 Results

We have operated on 30 patients since 2022 with this technique. We have 75% of satisfied patients who do not need any further surgery. The other 25% need to undergo surgery such as arthroscopy or shoulder prosthesis. For us, it is now our first line of therapy for patients with arthritis and painful shoulders with still a good range of motion.

Take-Home Message

Indication

Patient with surgery indications for the tenotomy of the biceps.

Arthrosis of the shoulder with still good mobility but the clinical aspect is more pain especially pain at night and during external rotation.

The patient must be informed of the major risk of Popeye deformity in post-op.

Contraindication

Patients that need open surgery:

Arthrosis in a young patient, a patient with a stiff shoulder.

Surgical Technique

(a) WALANT anesthesia 30/50 cc.
(b) Transverse view of the biceps tendon at the top of the groove when this one is flattening. The patient must be in neutral rotation.
(c) Find the best entry point with a 25-gauge needle on a transverse view of the biceps. The probe should be 2 cm distal from the anterior lateral aspect of the acromion. The needle should go straight under the tendon. The anesthesia can be improved if needed.
(d) Open the skin with a knife on 1.5 cm.
(e) Pass a Halstead forceps under the skin to free the fascia and perforate the sheet around the tendon.
(f) Then, pass the Halstead forceps beneath the cortex of the humeral bone and the muscle.
(g) Insert the beaver, and control on in-plane view the position of the beaver under the tendon and up the cortex. The beaver should be inserted on its lateral face to improve the ultrasound resolution.
(h) After 90° rotation, the sharp part of the knife is under the tendon. The cutting is realized with small movements up and down.
(i) Control the release with a Halstead forceps.

Postoperative care

(a) Pressure dressing for 48 h.
(b) No immobilization is needed.

Conclusion

Ultrasound release of the biceps tendon at the shoulder level is efficient in diminishing the pain in certain patients with shoulder arthrosis. The recovery is fast and without any immobilization. The risk of failure is 20/25% but without major complications and without cutting any bridge to other solutions.

Bibliography

1. Dufour M, Del Valle S. Les muscles. Maloine: Anatomie clinique des membres; 2017.
2. SOFCOT [Internet]. [cité 20 juin 2023]. La pathologie de la longue portion du biceps. Disponible sur: https://www.sofcot.fr/media/1350
3. Snyder GM, Mair SD, Lattermann C. Tendinopathy of the long head of the biceps. In: Maffulli N, editor. Medicine and sport science [Internet]. S. Karger AG, [cité 25 juin 2023]; 2012. p. 76–89. Disponible sur: https://www.karger.com/Article/FullText/328880.
4. Lalehzarian SP, Agarwalla A, Liu JN. Management of proximal biceps tendon pathology. WJO. 2022;13(1):36–57.
5. Nho SJ, Strauss EJ, Lenart BA, Provencher MT, Mazzocca AD, Verma NN, et al. Long head of the biceps tendinopathy: diagnosis and management: American Academy of Orthopaedic. Surgeon. 2010;18(11):645–56.
6. Wilk KE, Hooks TR. The painful long head of the biceps Brachii. Clin Sports Med. 2016;35(1):75–92.
7. Varacallo M, Mair SD. Proximal biceps tendinitis and tendinopathy. In: StatPearls [Internet]. Treasure Island (FL): StatPearls Publishing; 2023. [cité 25 juin 2023]. Disponible sur: http://www.ncbi.nlm.nih.gov/books/NBK533002/.
8. Di Benedetto P, Mancuso F, Tosolini L, Buttironi MM, Beltrame A, Causero A. Treatment options for massive rotator cuff tears: a narrative review. Acta Biomedica Atenei Parmensis. 2021;92(S3):e2021026.

9. Cuéllar A, Cuéllar A, Cuéllar R. Editorial commentary: shoulder biceps Tenodesis versus Tenotomy: both show good results and have different indications. Arthroscopy. 2022;38(6):1843–5.
10. Patel KV, Bravman J, Vidal A, Chrisman A, McCarty E. Biceps Tenotomy versus Tenodesis. Clin Sports Med. 2016;35(1):93–111.
11. Kooistra B, Gurnani N, Weening A, Van Deurzen D, Van Den Bekerom M. Tenotomy or Tenodesis for tendinopathy of the long head of the biceps Brachii: an updated systematic review and meta-analysis. Arthrosc Sports Med Rehabil. 2021;3(4):e1199–209.
12. Zhou P, Liu J, Deng X, Li Z. Biceps tenotomy versus tenodesis for lesions of the long head of the biceps tendon: a systematic review and meta-analysis of randomized controlled trials. Medicine. 2021;100(3):e23993.
13. Hsu AR, Ghodadra NS, Provencher CMT, Lewis PB, Bach BR. Biceps tenotomy versus tenodesis: a review of clinical outcomes and biomechanical results. J Shoulder Elb Surg. 2011;20(2):326–32.
14. SFA, Potel JF, Hulet C. L'arthroscopie. Elsevier Masson; 2015. p. 1384.
15. Fick B, Stover DW, Chimenti RL, Hall MM. The safety of ultrasound guided Tenotomy and debridement for upper and lower extremity tendinopathies: a retrospective study. Iowa Orthop J. 2021;41(2):82–90.
16. Lane D, Schiller T. Technique description: incisionless ultrasound-assisted biceps tenotomy in dogs. Open Vet J. 2021;10(4):457–64.
17. Esterline ML, Armbrust L, Roush JK. A comparison of palpation guided and ultrasound guided percutaneous biceps brachii tenotomy in dogs. Vet Comp Orthop Traumatol. 2005;18(3):135–9.
18. Marès O. L'échochirurgie du membre supérieur. Etat d'un art Sauramps Médical; 2021. p. 145.

18 Ultrasound-Guided Fasciotomy in Chronic Exertional Compartment Syndrome of the Forearm

Jean Michel Cognet

18.1 Introduction

Forearm chronic exertional compartment syndrome (FCECS) is a rare pathology that mainly affects musicians and athletes that perform repeated and prolonged forced grasping movements (motorcycling, rowing, mountain biking, windsurfing, etc.) [1–4]. These movements cause an increase in muscular volume between 20 and 30% [5, 6] in an inextensible compartment, raising intramuscular pressure (IMP) and lowering veinous circulation leading to ischemia and muscular edema.

FCECS etiology is poorly understood. A congenital anatomic predisposition has been hypothesized by certain authors [7, 8]. FCECS is bilateral in 70–100% of cases and predominantly affects young males [9]. It presents as cramps, beginning at the anteromedial aspect of the forearm before spreading to the whole forearm and can be accompanied by weakness and paresthesia [10]. Symptoms begin 5–10 min after begging of the effort and typically disappear in 15–30 min after cessation [11]. The diagnosis is made through the association of clinical signs and a pathological IMP. Unfortunately, this criterion is ill-defined and there is no consensus on the method of measurement or the pathological thresholds. Schoeffl et al. found IMPs of 36 mmHg in asymptomatic patients [12], whereas Ruyer et al. found 18% false negatives [13]. Rydholm et al. noted that IMP during exercise could increase six fold in cases of FCECS [14] and IMP on the symptomatic side returned to baseline slower than the asymptomatic side, corroborating *Barrera-Ochoa*'s hypothesis that delay to normalization of IMP could be more pertinent in the diagnosis of FCECS [11]. The multiple diagnostic criteria show the difficulty in finding a consensus [15, 16]. Pain rarely dissipates without the cessation of the causal activity [12]. Conservative treatment, albeit efficient in 50–80% of cases, often requires the cessation of the incriminating sport and remains difficult or even unacceptable for patients, even more so when surgical is efficient in 70–90% of patients [7, 12, 14].

18.2 Diagnosis

In the upper limb, it occurs essentially in motorcyclists practicing their sport in competition with several hours of training per week [17–19]. The engine size is also a factor, and it has been shown that moving from a 250 cc motorcycle to a 600 cc motorcycle increases the risk of exertional compartment syndrome. Other sports may be concerned: kayaking, water skiing, wind surfing, weight training, etc.

J. M. Cognet (✉)
Médipole, Bezannes, France

O. Marès et al. (eds.), *Ultrasound-Guided Limb Surgery*,
https://doi.org/10.1007/978-3-031-88679-9_18

The clinical presentation is characteristic with the onset of cramps 5–10 min after the beginning of the sport or almost always at the same time after the beginning of the effort: The patient often knows very well after how long he will start to feel discomfort and must stop. These cramps can be associated with paresthesias, which can lead to the suspicion of a compression of the median nerve in the carpal tunnel, knowing that the two pathologies are sometimes associated. There is also pain and weakness of the grip that can be dangerous when riding a motorcycle. Stopping the sport activity usually leads to the disappearance of the clinical symptomatology in 15–30 min. Patients are able to reproduce their symptomatology by repeated forearm contraction movements for 3–4 min.

The diagnosis is made based on the measurement of the pressure of the lodges at rest and during exercise (Fig. 18.1). A pressure > 15 mm Hg at rest, 30 mm Hg during exercise, or 20 mm Hg 5 min after stopping the activity is considered pathological. There have been some results with the use of magnetic resonance imaging in FCECS, showing edema surrounding the flexor digitorum superficialis and profundus when compared with asymptomatic individuals; however, this is a nonspecific finding and can be found in other pathological conditions and therefore has not been consistently reliable [20].

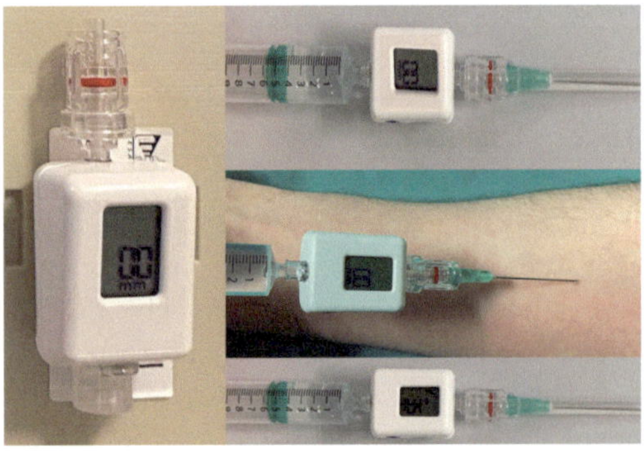

Fig. 18.1 Intramuscular pressure (IMP) measurement. A measurement gauge is connected to a syringe with saline solution on one side and an 18-guage needle on the other. The system is purged with saline and then IMP is measured. Diastolic pressure is then subtracted for the final measurement

18.3 Treatment

Treatment of FCECS is indicated if there is typical clinical symptomatology and positive compartment pressure measurement.

Medical management has been proposed [13], involving a modification and/or improvement of movement, and often depends on the sports environment and the doctor in charge of monitoring the athlete. If there is no improvement after 3 months of medical treatment, surgery may be proposed. If medical treatment fails and the patient does not wish to undergo surgery, the pain persists, eventually leading to cessation of sporting activity [7, 12, 14].

Two surgical techniques are currently used for the management of stress compartment syndromes: open and percutaneous surgery.

18.3.1 Open Surgery

An incision is made on the anterior aspect of the forearm from the medial condyle in the direction of the radial styloid over a distance of about 20 cm. An arched incision can also be made to avoid the occurrence of skin flaps. It is not necessary to extend the incision to the wrist. This wide approach allows the superficial and deep compartment of the forearm to be freed. As a rule, this is a fasciotomy. Fasciectomy is not necessary, except in the case of revision for recurrence.

The success rate of open fasciotomy is close to 90%, but it is not free of complications related to the size of the incision: skin disunion, enlargement of the scar with time, scar fibrosis that may reproduce compartment syndrome, etc.

18.3.2 Percutaneous Surgery

The purpose of this surgery is to reduce scarring. We will only deal here with true percutaneous surgery with endoscopic or ultrasound assistance.

18.3.2.1 Fasciotomy Under Endoscopic Control of the Anterior Compartment

This technique was reported by Fontes et al [1] For him, it is not necessary to perform open surgery in FCECS for several reasons: The existence of a deep fascia separating the superficial and deep planes remains debated; the release of the anterior compartment leads to a decrease in pressure in the adjacent compartments; the opening of the skin has no additional beneficial effect (contrary to the acute compartment syndrome) and entails a risk of unsightly scarring and skin adhesions, sources of potential recurrence.

Other authors have reported their experience with the endoscopic technique in recent years with excellent results [2, 21, 22]. Marwan et al. published a review of the literature in 2021, which found a success rate of 98.4% for the endoscopic technique [9].

18.3.2.2 Personal Technique: Fasciotomy Under Ultrasound Assistance

Surgery is performed under regional or general anesthesia (in cases of bilateral surgery), supine with the use of an arm tourniquet at 250 mmHg and an arm table.

Only the anterior superficial compartment is opened, and the technique is similar to the blind percutaneous "mini-open" approach described by Croutzet et al [16].

A line is drawn on the anterior forearm from the medial humeral epicondyle to the radial styloid. On this line four marks are made every 6–7 cm.

Two transversal skin incisions are made, the antebrachial fascia exposed and incised. Blunt-tipped scissors are used to free the fascia from surrounding structures on its superficial and deep aspects at each incision, proximally and distally (Fig. 18.2).

The fasciotomy is performed using a dedicated scalpel (Kemis H3 knife, Newclip) under US visualization (3–16 MHz linear probe, HS40 US, Samsung) (Figs. 18.3 and 18.4).

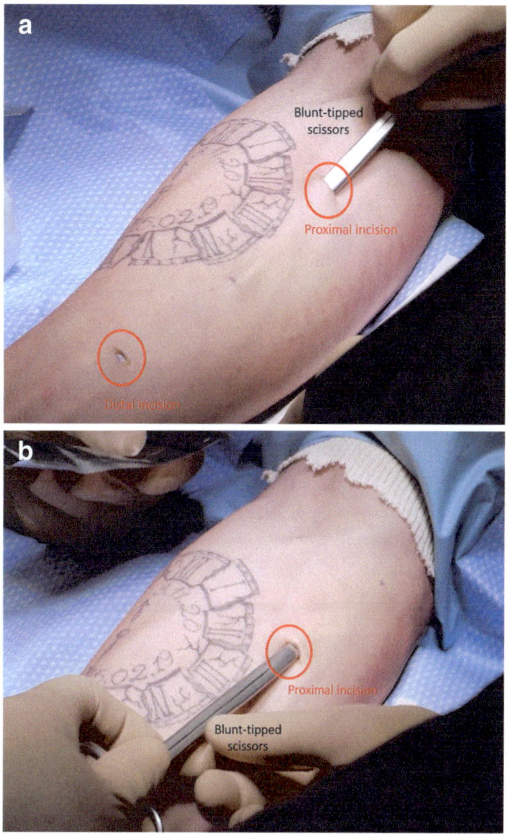

Fig. 18.2 Blunt-tipped scissors were used to free the fascia from surrounding structures on its superficial and deep aspects at each incision, distally (**a**) and proximally (**b**)

The scissors are then used under ultrasound guidance to verify the fasciotomy is complete by freely passing between the muscle and subcutaneous tissue (Fig. 18.5).

Tourniquet is deflated prior to closure. No drainage is used; however a compressive silicone tubing is applied for 72 h. Patient is encouraged to mobilize fingers and use forearm for daily activities. A quick return to activities is encouraged (2 weeks) in order to prevent fibrous adherences.

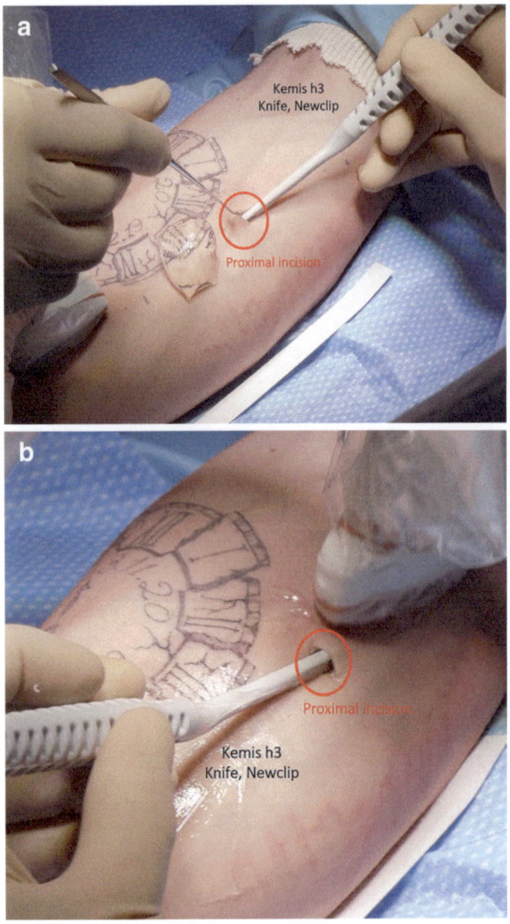

Fig. 18.3 The fasciotomy is done under US guidance, distally (**a**) and proximally (**b**) for each incision

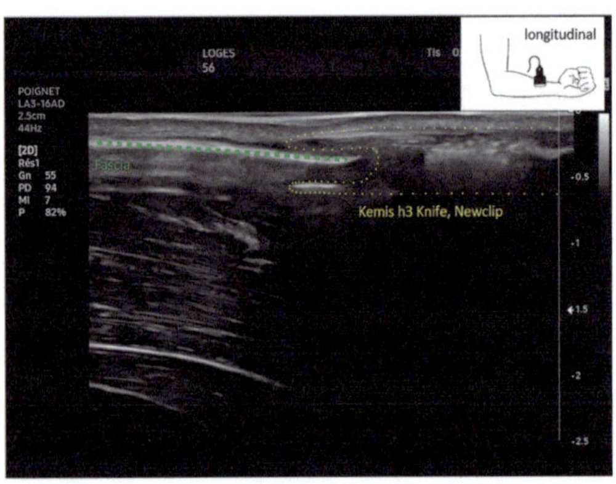

Fig. 18.4 US guidance during the fasciotomy (longitudinal view)

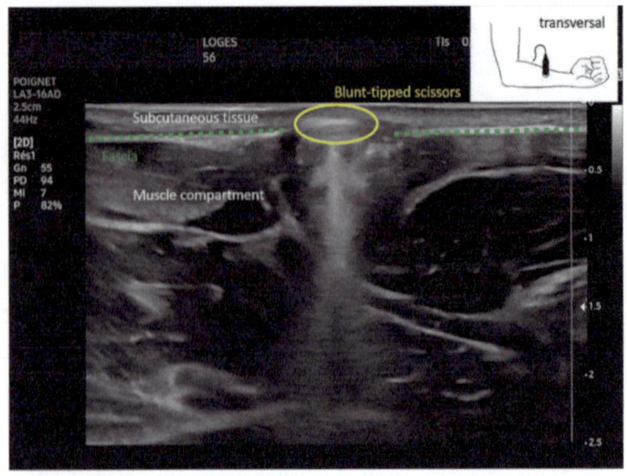

Fig. 18.5 At the end of the fasciotomy, blunt-tipped scissors are inserted and passed from the muscle to the subcutaneous tissue under US control (transversal view) confirming the complete fasciotomy

Take-Home Messages

Indication

Clinical symptomatology

And positive compartment pressure measurement

And no improvement after 3 months of medical treatment

Contraindication: None

Surgical Technique

(a) Regional or general anesthesia
(b) Line is drawn from the medial humeral epicondyle to the radial styloid. On this line four marks are made every 6–7 cm. Two transversal skin incisions are made
(c) The antebrachial fascia is exposed and incised. Blunt-tipped scissors are used to free the fascia from surrounding structures on its superficial and deep aspects at each incision, proximally and distally
(d) Dedicated scalpel (Kemis H3 knife, Newclip)

Postoperative care

Pressure dressing for 72 h

No mobility restriction

Bibliography

1. Fontes D, Clement R, Roure P. Endoscopic aponeurotomy for chronic exertional compartmental syndrome of the forearm: report of 41 cases. Chir Main. 2003;22(4):186–96.
2. Pozzi A, Pivato G, Kask K, Susini F, Pegoli L. Single portal endoscopic treatment for chronic exertional compartment syndrome of the forearm. Tech Hand Up Extrem Surg. 2014;18:153–6.
3. Harrison JWK, Thomas P, Aster A, Wilkes G, Hayton MJ. Chronic exertional compartment syndrome of the forearm in elite rowers: a technique for mini-open fasciotomy and a report of six cases. Hand (NY). 2013;8:450–3.
4. Liu B, Barrazueta G, Ruchelsman DE. Chronic exertional compartment syndrome in athletes. J Hand Surg Am. 2017;42:917–23.
5. Wright JM, Bogoch ER, Hastings DE. The "occult" compartment syndrome. J Trauma. 1989:29133–4.
6. Rorabeck CH, Mc Nab MB. The pathophysiology of the anterior tibial compartmental syndrome. Clin Orthop. 1975;113:52–7.
7. García Mata S, Hidalgo Ovejero A, Martinez Grande M. Bilateral, chronic exertional compartment syndrome of the forearm in two brothers. Clin J Sport Med. 1999;9(2):91–9.
8. Wasilewski SA, Asdourian PL. Bilateral chronic exertional compartment syndromes of forearm in an adolescent athlete: Case report and review of literature. Am J Sports Med. 1991;19:665–7.
9. Marwan Y, Addar A, Algarni N, Algarni N, Burman M, Martineau PA. Endoscopic fasciotomy for chronic exertional compartment syndrome of the forearm: Systematic review of outcomes and complications. World J Orthop. 2021;12(5):320–8.
10. Boody AR, Wongworawat MD. Accuracy in the measurement of compartment pressures: a comparison of three commonly used devices. J Bone Joint Surg Am. 2005;87(11):2415–22.
11. Barrera-Ochoa S, Haddad S, Correa-Vazquez E, Segura JF, Gil E, Lluch A, et al. Surgical decompression of exertional compartment syndrome of the forearm in professional motorcycling racers: comparative long-term results of wide open versus mini-open fasciotomy. Clin J Sport Med. 2016;26:108–14.
12. Brown JS, Wheeler PC, Boyd KT, Barnes MR, Allen MJ. Chronic exertional compartment syndrome of the forearm: a case series of 12 patients treated with fasciotomy. J Hand Surg Eur. 2011;36(5):413–9.
13. Hutchinson MR, Ireland ML. Common compartment syndromes in athletes. Treatment and rehabilitation. Sports Med. 1994;17(3):200–8.
14. Guerzider Regas I, Pluvy I, Tuphe P, Sakek F, Fuchs B, Haight H, et al. Long term functional outcomes after minimally invasive surgical decompression in upper limb chronic exertional compartment syndrome in 30 patients. Hand Surg Rehabil. 2021;40(1):32–9.
15. Zandi H, Bell S. Results of compartment decompression in chronic forearm compartment syndrome: six case presentations. Br J Sports Med. 2005;39:e35.
16. Croutzet P, Chassat R, Masmejean EH. Mini-invasive surgery for chronic exertional compartment syndrome of the forearm: a new technique. Tech Hand Up Extrem Surg. 2009;13(3):137–40.
17. Humpherys J, Lum Z, Cohen J. Diagnosis and treatment of chronic exertional compartment syndrome of the forearm in motocross riders. JBJS Rev. 2018;6(1):e3.
18. Pedowitz RA, Hargens AR, Mubarak SJ, Gershuni DH. Modified criteria for the objective diagnosis of chronic compartment syndrome of the leg. Am J Sports Med. 1990;18(1):35–40.
19. Regas I, Pluvy I, Sakek F, Tuphe P, Ortega P, Guinchard B, et al. Epidemiology of upper limb chronic exertional compartment syndrome (CECS) in the French Motorcycle Federation racers: Results of a national questionnaire-based study. Hand Surg Rehabil. 2021;40(3):268–76.
20. Kumar PR, Jenkins JPR, Hodgson SP. Bilateral chronic exertional compartment syndrome of the dorsal part of the forearm: the role of magnetic resonance imaging in diagnosis: a case report. J Bone Joint Surg Am. 2003;85(8):1557–9.
21. Pegoli L, Pozzi A, Pivato G. Endoscopic single approach forearm fasciotomy for chronic exertional compartment syndrome: long term follow-up. J Hand Surg Asian-Pacific Vol. 2016;21(1):8–12.
22. Miller EA, Cobb AL, Cobb TK. Endoscopic fascia release for forearm chronic exertional compartment syndrome: case report and surgical technique. Hand (New York). 2017;12(5):Np58-np61

Part VI

Thigh

19 Ultrasound-Guided Iliotibial Band Release

Remy Coulomb, Valentin Cascales, Olivier Mares, and Pascal Kouyoumdjian

19.1 Introduction

External snapping hip (ESH) or lateral coxa saltans is an extra-articular phenomenon involving the passage of the iliotibial band (ITB) over the greater trochanter prominence. This sudden passage is often audible during hip flexion or active extension and can be painful [1]. Whether voluntary or not, this phenomenon is exacerbated by the thickening of the posterior part of the ITB or the anterior margin of the gluteus maximus muscle [2]. LHS dominantly affects young women engaged in sports with repetitive hip movements [2].

19.2 Diagnosis

The diagnosis of ESH is primarily clinical. It is essential to assess whether it is associated with lateral hip pain, which may indicate pre-trochanteric bursitis or gluteal pathology [2]. Pain is a prognostic factor for poorer therapeutic outcomes. Lateral snapping can be confirmed by ultrasound (US) through reproduction during dynamic examination. Radiography is performed to rule out architectural abnormalities or additional joint issues. In cases of persistent pain or atypical presentations, magnetic resonance imaging (MRI) can help exclude gluteal pathology [2, 3].

19.3 Treatment

19.3.1 Personal Technique

The described technique draws inspiration from the endoscopic surgical technique outlined by Zini et al. [4]. It involves a single posterior incision along the lateral prominence of the greater trochanter, providing access to the ITB. The ITB is then released from posterior to anterior direction, avoiding iatrogenic sciatic nerve injury, using a disposable Kemis© knife known for its application in median nerve carpal tunnel release.

The patient is positioned in lateral position, opposite to the lesion. A lateral support or leg spacer aids in ITB relaxation. The entire hip is draped to mobilize it and replicate snapping. Ultrasound examination of the hip is performed using a linear multifrequency transducer (5–12 MHz) in longitudinal and transverse planes to identify relevant anatomical structures: the lateral facet of the greater trochanter, ischium, sciatic nerve, anterior border of the gluteus maximus, ITB, tensor fascia lata, and lateral femoral cutaneous nerve.

Local anesthesia with 20 cc of 1% xylocaine plus epinephrine is administered under ultrasound guidance, adjacent to deep and superficial parts

R. Coulomb (✉) · V. Cascales · O. Mares
P. Kouyoumdjian
Department of Traumatology and Orthopedic, University Hospital Nîmes, Nîmes, France

O. Marès et al. (eds.), *Ultrasound-Guided Limb Surgery*,
https://doi.org/10.1007/978-3-031-88679-9_19

of the ITB, to separate layers by hydrodissection (Fig. 19.1). This process enhances echogenicity, aided by superficial positioning of major structures and bony contrast of the greater trochanter.

With ultrasound guidance, the transducer is positioned transversely to the most prominent part of the greater trochanter, distal to its end. The thickened posterior part of the ITB is identified, and a 5 mm skin incision is made near the posterior edge of the greater trochanter. A curved Halsted forceps is passed through this incision to confirm release of deep and superficial layers of the ITB (Fig. 19.2). The disposable Kemis knife is then inserted under ultrasound guidance until it engages the posterior part of the ITB between its jaws, at its junction with the anterior edge of the gluteus maximus muscle. A transverse cut is made across the width of the greater trochanter, with the anterior limit of the section being the posterior border of the tensor fascia lata muscle (Fig. 19.3). The knife curvature allows for sectioning of the posterior half of the ITB, followed by a 180-degree rotation downward for sectioning of the anterior half. At the procedure's completion, ITB release is re-evaluated under ultrasound guidance. The curved Halsted forceps is used to probe the deep part of the ITB along the entire width of the greater trochanter. If fibers remain, the knife is used for further cutting if necessary. The advantage is to realize this procedure under local to assess the complete disappearance of the snapping when the ITB section is sufficient.

This technique allows us to realize an "à la carte" procedure under awake patients until the snapping disappears. Post-operative dressing is done by the patient, and active motion is encouraged the day after surgery. Active training is delayed by 1 month.

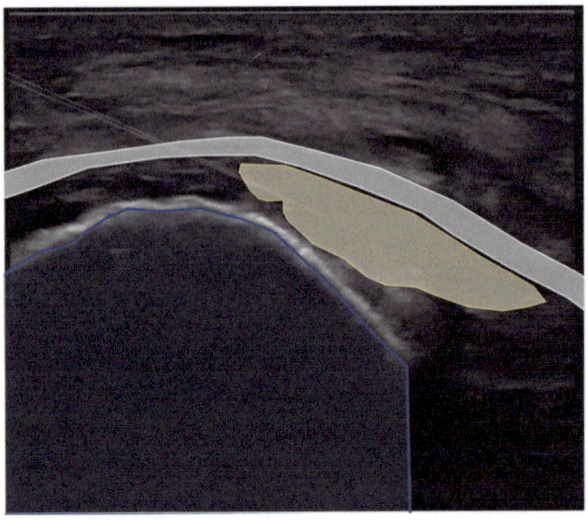

Fig. 19.1 Hydrodissection on a transverse view: the needle is under the fascia

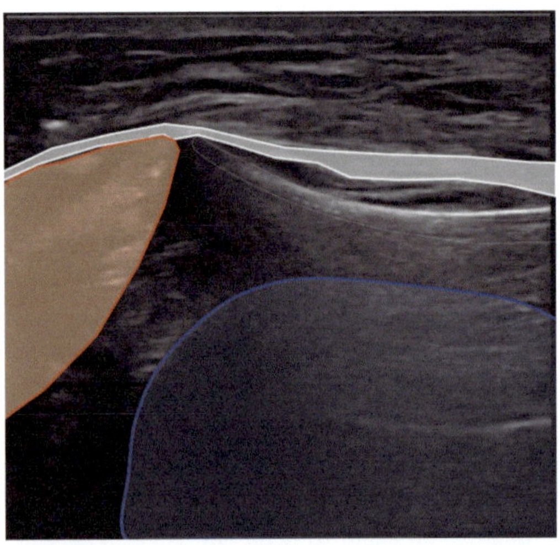

Fig. 19.2 Transverse view with the Halsted forceps under the fascia lata

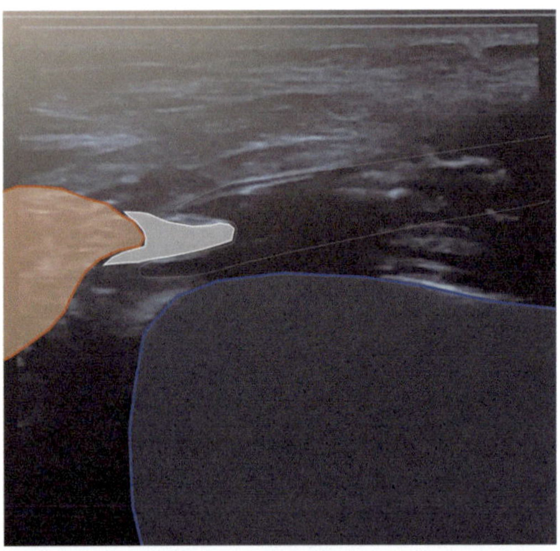

Fig. 19.3 Section on a transverse view of the fascia lata with the Kemis knife

Take-Home Message

Indication

Lateral hip snapping

Contraindication

Gluteal pathology

Surgical Technique

(a) Local anesthesia with 20 cc Rapido-Epinephrine 1% administered at the posterior part of the greater trochanter, adjacent to the anterior border of the gluteus maximus, superficial and deep injection of the ITB.
(b) Control ITB limits with a US transverse view and mark the anterior border of the gluteus maximus and posterior of the fascia lata.
(c) Make a 5 mm skin incision with an N°11 blade orthogonal to the leg axis.
(d) Perform subcutaneous dissection with a Halsted forceps. Pierce the retinaculum. Control instrument position on transverse and longitudinal views.
(e) Introduce the knife. Verify on transverse and longitudinal views that only the lower blade is under the ITB.
(f) Gently push the knife anteriorly (holding your probe horizontally) to the most prominent point of the greater trochanter.
(g) Rotate the knife 180° and verify on transverse and longitudinal views that only the upper blade is under the ITB.
(h) Gently push the knife anteriorly to the posterior border of the tensor fascia lata.
(i) Check complete freeing of the ITB section using a Halsted forceps.

Postoperative care

Pressure dressing for 24 h

No mobility restriction

References

1. Yen YM, Lewis CL, Kim IJ. Understanding and treating the snapping hip. Sports Med Arthrosc. 2015;23:194–9.
2. Sunil Kumar KH, Rawal J, Nakano N, Sarmento A, Khanduja V. Pathogenesis and contemporary diagnoses for lateral hip pain: a scoping review. Knee Surg Sports Traumatol Arthrosc. 2021;29:2408–16. https://doi.org/10.1007/s00167-020-06354-1. Epub 2020 Dec 19
3. Walker P, Ellis E, Scofield J, Kongchum T, Sherman WF, Kaye AD. Snapping hip syndrome: a comprehensive update. Orthop Rev. 2021;13:25088.
4. Zini R, Munegato D, De Benedetto M, Carraro A, Bigoni M. Endoscopic iliotibial band release in snapping hip. Hip Int. 2013;23:225–32.

20 Ultrasound-Guided Fasciotomy for Chronic Exertional Compartment Syndrome

Guillaume Prado and Julien Beldame

20.1 Introduction

Chronic exertional compartment syndrome (CECS) is a condition characterized by increased pressure within the muscle compartments. This syndrome is most commonly observed in athletes who engage in repetitive impact activities such as running, jumping, or motocross, leading to recurrent pain that may limit sporting activities. This affection compromises microcirculation causing tissue ischemia and nerve dysfunction [1]. The epidemiology of this pathology is underestimated, in both leg and forearm compartment syndromes. The condition often manifests in individuals between the ages of 20 and 30, with no predominance between men and women [2]. In the lower limb, this pathology affects the anterior leg compartment in 48% of cases and the deep posterior compartment in 40%. There are few data in the literature concerning the forearm [3].

G. Prado (✉)
Cabinet de médicine du Sport de Medicity, Saint-Malo, France

J. Beldame
Institut de la Cheville et du Pied Amiens, Polyclinique de Picardie, Amiens, France

Institut de la Cheville et du Pied Paris, Paris, France

20.2 Diagnostic Approach

The diagnosis of anterior compartment syndrome is primarily clinical but requires confirmation through compartment pressure testing, which remains the gold standard. Symptoms typically include a cramping sensation and bulging in the affected compartment, exacerbated by exercise and relieved by rest. The presence of muscle hernias is often observed. Patients describe a progressive increase in pain during exercise, which promptly diminishes upon cessation of the activity.

Compartment pressures should be measured both at rest and immediately after exercise to accurately diagnose CECS. Pressures exceeding 15 mmHg at rest, or 30 mmHg post-exercise, or greater than 20 mmHg after the first 5 min after exercise cessation, are indicative of CECS [4]. Additionally, advanced imaging techniques like MRI or scintigraphy can assist in ruling out other pathologies such as stress fractures or muscle hernias [5–7].

20.3 Treatment

20.3.1 Conservative Management

According to the latest Clinical Consensus on Diagnosis and Treatment of Patients with Chronic Exertional Compartment Syndrome of the Leg, it

O. Marès et al. (eds.), *Ultrasound-Guided Limb Surgery*,
https://doi.org/10.1007/978-3-031-88679-9_20

is essential that gait retraining and cessation of provoking activities are valuable components of a conservative treatment program. The panel considered guidance and treatment by a physical therapist, shoe modifications, or botulinum injections not essential for a conservative treatment regimen, but rather as potential additions depending on patient needs [8].

20.3.2 Surgical Management

Recent advancements in surgical techniques for the treatment of chronic exertional compartment syndrome have focused on minimally invasive methods to reduce recovery time and improve functional outcomes [3, 9]. The arthroscopic assisted mini-incisional fasciotomy technique has advantages such as early rehabilitation and good cosmetic appearance [10]. However, this technique is limited by the length of the canula (requiring three or four incisions from the proximal to the distal part of the leg) and represents a risk for the superficial peroneal nerve who is not controlled during the procedure [11]. Superficial peroneal nerve injury is the most common iatrogenic complication of surgical fasciotomy procedure up to 8% of the cases treated [11]. Ultrasound-guided fasciotomy is an innovative approach that enhances the precision of the surgical intervention while minimizing collateral tissue damage, skin incision, and superficial peroneal nerve injury.

20.4 Ultrasound-Guided Fasciotomy

20.4.1 Step-by-Step Procedure

1. *Preoperative planning and patient preparation:* Prior to the procedure, a comprehensive ultrasound examination is conducted to map out the anatomy of the affected compartment and to plan the fasciotomy incision. The patient is positioned supine, with the leg slightly elevated and internally rotated to optimize ultrasound visibility and surgeon access. Ultrasound can easily identify vascular and neural elements such as the superficial fibular nerve in the anterior compartment of the leg. Anatomical possible lesions were venous and small subcutaneous arteries and superficial peroneal nerve. Subcutaneous vessels are easily noted by ultrasound during procedure. Small saphenous pedicle is the most important structure. Superficial fibular nerve is controlled on the distal third part of the leg (forming a honeycomb pattern), on the anterior part of the fibula when the nerve cross through the aponeurosis (Figs. 20.1 and 20.2). This level is located from 10 to 15 cm proximally to the tip of the fibula. This point of cross section is drawing on the skin and branches of the nerve are following on the subcutaneous tissues. Different anatomical variation existed into subcutaneous tissues sometime with division onto two branches on the distal part of the leg.
2. *Anesthesia:* Local anesthesia or WALLANT are typically employed, which not only ensures patient comfort but also aids in muscle relaxation, facilitating a more straightforward surgical approach. Anesthesia is also used to prepare localization of the section and make hydrodissection of anatomical structure. Most part of the hydrodissection must be done into the subcutaneous tissue between the aponeurosis and superficial peroneal nerve branches.
3. *Ultrasound-guided access:* Using a high-resolution ultrasound machine, the surgeon visualizes the fascia of the anterior compart-

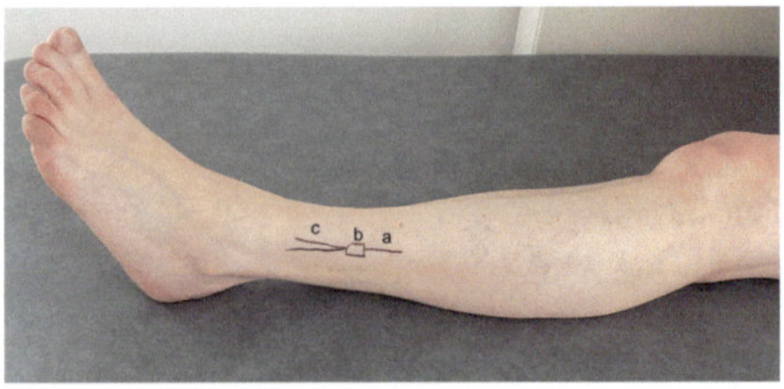

Fig. 20.1 Skin drawing of the superficial fibular nerve passing from anterior muscle compartment to the subcutaneous tissues

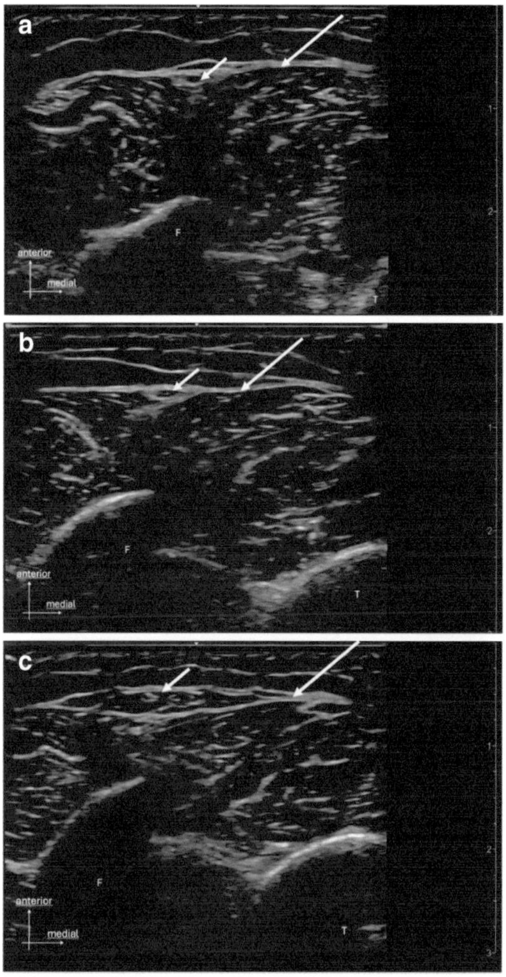

Fig. 20.2 Ultrasound "out-of-plane" image. (**a**) SFN into the anterior muscle compartment, (**b**) SFN just before his crossing, (**c**) SFN into subcutaneous tissues and its bifurcation. Long arrow, the anterior fascia; short arrow, superficial fibular nerve (SFN); F, fibula; T, tibia

ment. Real-time imaging guides the insertion of the surgical instruments, ensuring accurate placement and minimizing the risk of damaging nearby structures. Depending on the cutting instrument (retrograde or anterograde knife, design, length, etc.), only one incision can be made on the middle part of the leg, allowing access to the proximal part of the aponeurosis by a retrograde section and by an anterograde section on the distal part. Sealing the entry point with Betadine gel™ prevents air bubbles from entering and distorting the ultrasound image. A skin portal 5 or 6 cm proximal to the cross section of the superficial peroneal nerve is easier for a better handling of the cutting knife (on the distal part of the leg that required prevent lesion of nerve branches), compared to a proximal portal who need to work under many centimeters of subcutaneous tissues before arriving to the danger zone of the cross section of the peroneal nerve.

4. *Fasciotomy:* Specialized fasciotomy instruments or a scalpel is introduced through a small incision under continuous ultrasound guidance. The fascia is then carefully incised longitudinally, ensuring complete release of the compartment. The length and depth of the incision are constantly monitored on the ultrasound screen to confirm adequate decompression.
5. *Closure and postoperative care:* The incision is typically closed with minimal suturing, if necessary. Postoperative care includes limb elevation, compression, and gradual mobilization. Rehabilitation begins within a few days to maintain range of motion and gradually reintroduce load-bearing activities.

20.5 Conclusion

Ultrasound-guided fasciotomy represents a significant advancement in the treatment of anterior compartment syndrome, offering a targeted approach that maximizes therapeutic efficacy while minimizing procedural invasiveness and recovery time. This technique, though still emerging, promises a quicker return to activity with reduced complications, representing a substantial improvement over traditional surgical methods. Further studies and long-term follow-ups are necessary to fully establish its benefits and procedural optimizations.

Take-Home Messages

Indication

Patients with clinical symptoms and objectively elevated lower extremity compartment pressure when conservative treatment has failed

Surgical Technique

- Prior comprehensive ultrasound examination
- WALANT anesthesia
- Transverse view of the insertion of the plantar fascia at the calcaneum level
- One portal at the middle part of the leg: 5–6 cm proximal to the point where the superficial peronal nerve pierces the superfical aponeurosis
- Proximal retrograde liberation and distal anterograde liberatión from the skin portal access. Under continuous ultrasound guidance

Postoperative care

- Limb elevation and pressure dressing for 48 h
- Rehabilitation starts within few days

References

1. Edmundsson D, Toolanen G, Thornell LE, Stål P. Evidence for low muscle capillary supply as a pathogenic factor in chronic compartment syndrome. Scand J Med Sci Sports. 2010;20(6):805–13.
2. Rothman R, Berke C, Jivanelli B, Casey E, Cheng J. Sex and gender differences in lower limb chronic exertional compartment syndrome: a systematic review. Phys Sportsmed. 2024;52(1):1–11.
3. Turnipseed WD. Diagnosis and management of chronic compartment syndrome. Surgery. 2002;132(4):613–7. discussion 617–619
4. Pedowitz RA, Hargens AR, Mubarak SJ, Gershuni DH. Modified criteria for the objective diagnosis of chronic compartment syndrome of the leg. Am J Sports Med. 1990;18(1):35–40.
5. Amendola A, Rorabeck CH, Vellett D, Vezina W, Rutt B, Nott L. The use of magnetic resonance imaging in exertional compartment syndromes. Am J Sports Med. 1990;18(1):29–34.
6. Hayes AA, Bower GD, Pitstock KL. Chronic (exertional) compartment syndrome of the legs diagnosed with thallous chloride scintigraphy. J Nucl Med Off Publ Soc Nucl Med. 1995;36(9):1618–24.
7. Takebayashi S, Takazawa H, Sasaki R, Miki H, Soh R, Nishimura J. Chronic exertional compartment syndrome in lower legs: localization and follow-up with thallium-201 SPECT imaging. J Nucl Med Off Publ Soc Nucl Med [Internet]. 1 juin 1997 [cité 1 mai 2024]; Disponible sur: https://www.semanticscholar.org/paper/Chronic-exertional-compartment-syndrome-in-lower-Takebayashi-Takazawa/3a16321958febb0bae3e624d9ee24ae266e7c110
8. Vogels S, Ritchie ED, van der Burg BLSB, Scheltinga MRM, Zimmermann WO, Hoencamp R. Clinical consensus on diagnosis and treatment of patients with chronic exertional compartment syndrome of the leg: a Delphi analysis. Sports Med Auckl Nz. 2022;52(12):3055–64.
9. Schiavi P, Gondolini G, Gandolfi CE, Guardoli L, Vaienti E, Zasa M. Mini-open surgical fasciotomy for chronic exertional compartment syndrome of the forearm in professional motorcycling adolescents. Clin J Sport Med Off J Can Acad Sport Med. 2020;30(6):e225–30.
10. Sebik A, Doğan A. A technique for arthroscopic fasciotomy for the chronic exertional tibialis anterior compartment syndrome. Knee Surg Sports Traumatol Arthrosc Off J ESSKA. 2008;16(5):531–4.
11. de Bruijn JA, van Zantvoort APM, Hundscheid HPH, Hoogeveen AR, Teijink JAW, Scheltinga MR. Superficial peroneal nerve injury risk during a semiblind fasciotomy for anterior chronic exertional compartment syndrome of the leg: an anatomical and clinical study. Foot Ankle Int. 2019;40(3):343–51.

21 Achilles Tendon Lengthening

G. Prado, R. Sacco, and J. Beldame

21.1 Introduction

The triceps surae, a muscular group occupying the superficial-posterior compartment of the leg, consists of the gastrocnemius, soleus, and plantaris muscles, collectively forming the gastrocnemius-soleus complex. The plantaris is present in up to 90% of cases [1].

Achilles tendon lengthening was initially performed to alleviate acquired plantar flexion contracture resulting from cerebral palsy in the pediatric population. More recently, numerous authors [2–5] have reported the prevalence of gastrocnemius contracture in patients with symptomatic midfoot or forefoot pathologies, including metatarsalgia, Morton foot deformity, posterior tibial tendon insufficiency, and plantar fasciitis.

The clinical diagnosis of gastrocnemius retraction (GR) relies on the Silfverskiold maneuver to distinguish gastrocnemius equinus from gastrocnemius-soleus equinus [6]. According to DiGiovanni et al. [2], GR is defined by passive ankle joint dorsiflexion of less than 5° with the knee extended for gastrocnemius equinus and less than 10° with the knee flexed for gastrocnemius-soleus equinus. Other authors consider GR as less than 10° of passive ankle dorsiflexion with the knee both flexed and extended [7].

21.2 Treatment

Various surgical techniques are available for releasing the gastrocnemius-soleus complex [8], with a progressive lengthening effect in a proximal to distal direction. The lengthening of the gastrocnemius-soleus complex is categorized into five levels [1, 9]:

Level 5: between proximal insertions and the common tendon of the medial and lateral gastrocnemius

Level 4: at the level of the medial and lateral bellies of the gastrocnemius

Level 3: at the tendinous zone between the beginning of the gastrocnemius common tendon to the common tendon with the soleus

G. Prado
Cabinet de Médicine du Sport de Medicity, Saint-Malo, France

R. Sacco
Centre Hospitalier de Rouen Universitaire de Rouen, Rouen, France

J. Beldame (✉)
Institut de la Cheville et du Pied Amiens, Polyclinique de Picardie, Amiens, France

Institut de la Cheville et du Pied Paris, Paris, France

O. Marès et al. (eds.), *Ultrasound-Guided Limb Surgery*,
https://doi.org/10.1007/978-3-031-88679-9_21

Level 2: from the common aponeurosis (gastrocnemius and soleus) to the end of the soleus muscle on the anterior part
Level 1: the tendinous area (calcaneal tendon)

Original techniques have undergone modifications to prevent complications (sural nerve injury), improve postoperative care and physiotherapy, decrease the size of skin incision, and minimize the risk of Achilles tendon rupture [10–13].

Achilles tendon lengthening (level 1), even though percutaneous procedures [10] or ultrasound control [14], exposes a risk of tendon rupture, needing non-weight bearing and postoperative immobilization. For these reasons they are reserved for severe neurological equinus.

Proximal and intermediate releases (from levels 2 to 5) are increasingly utilized, as they can be performed simultaneously with distal foot and ankle procedures. Postoperative management after gastrocnemius-soleus lengthening remains unchanged, as it does not require immobilization, allowing immediate full weight bearing. Moreover, lengthening at levels 2, 3, and 4 can be performed with the patient in a supine position. Only lengthening at level 1 must be performed in the prone position [15].

To simplify the operative technique and outcomes, endoscopic techniques have been developed (except for level 1) [16, 17] (Table 21.1).

For novice sonographers, ultrasound can primarily identify the height and position of the skin incision [18], avoiding uncertainty related to the variable morphology of patients. Ultrasound guidance is also an effective technique to prevent sural nerve injury: Preoperative ultrasound identification with skin marking allows for adapted skin incision.

Depending on the procedure, the level of lengthening, and portal incision, cutting instruments could be a needle (used perpendicular to the aponeurosis) or an anterograde/retrograde hook knife (used in the axis of the aponeurosis). Hook knife elongations are preferred (even if specific instruments are lacking) as they produce clean, complete, and longitudinal cuts, while needles may result in incomplete microsections with possible lesions of more superficial or deeper tissues.

For experienced sonographers, ultrasound can be used for a full ultrasound lengthening procedure. Only a few authors have described these types of procedures because they require sonographic experience and adapted cutting instruments. The localization, thickness, width, and shape of the gastrocnemius-soleus complex vary significantly between levels 1 and 5 (Fig. 21.1).

In level 1, a small blade or needles can be used for cutting the entire thickness of the tendon during a percutaneous procedure with a partial hemisection at different levels [10]. These procedures can be performed as an office procedure with local anesthesia [19].

At level 5, the procedure is possible under local anesthesia, but sedation is often necessary due to the richly innervated location of the release. Moreover, the medial gastrocnemius aponeurosis is located relatively deep under

Table 21.1 Ultrasound surgery

Villanueva et al. [20]	Proximal recession of the medial gastrocnemius	Anatomical study ($n = 16$) + 23 cases patients (no tourniquet and local anesthesia + sedation)	Hook knife
Iborra Marcos et al. [21]	Proximal recession of the medial gastrocnemius	Anatomical study ($n = 8$)	Needle
Moroni et al. [22]	Lengthening of the anterior gastrocnemius aponeurosis	Anatomical study ($n = 10$)	Hook knife
Villanueva et al. [23]	Lengthening of common aponeurosis between gastrocnemius and soleus	Anatomical study ($n = 22$) + 25 cases patients (no tourniquet and local anesthesia + sedation)	Hook knife

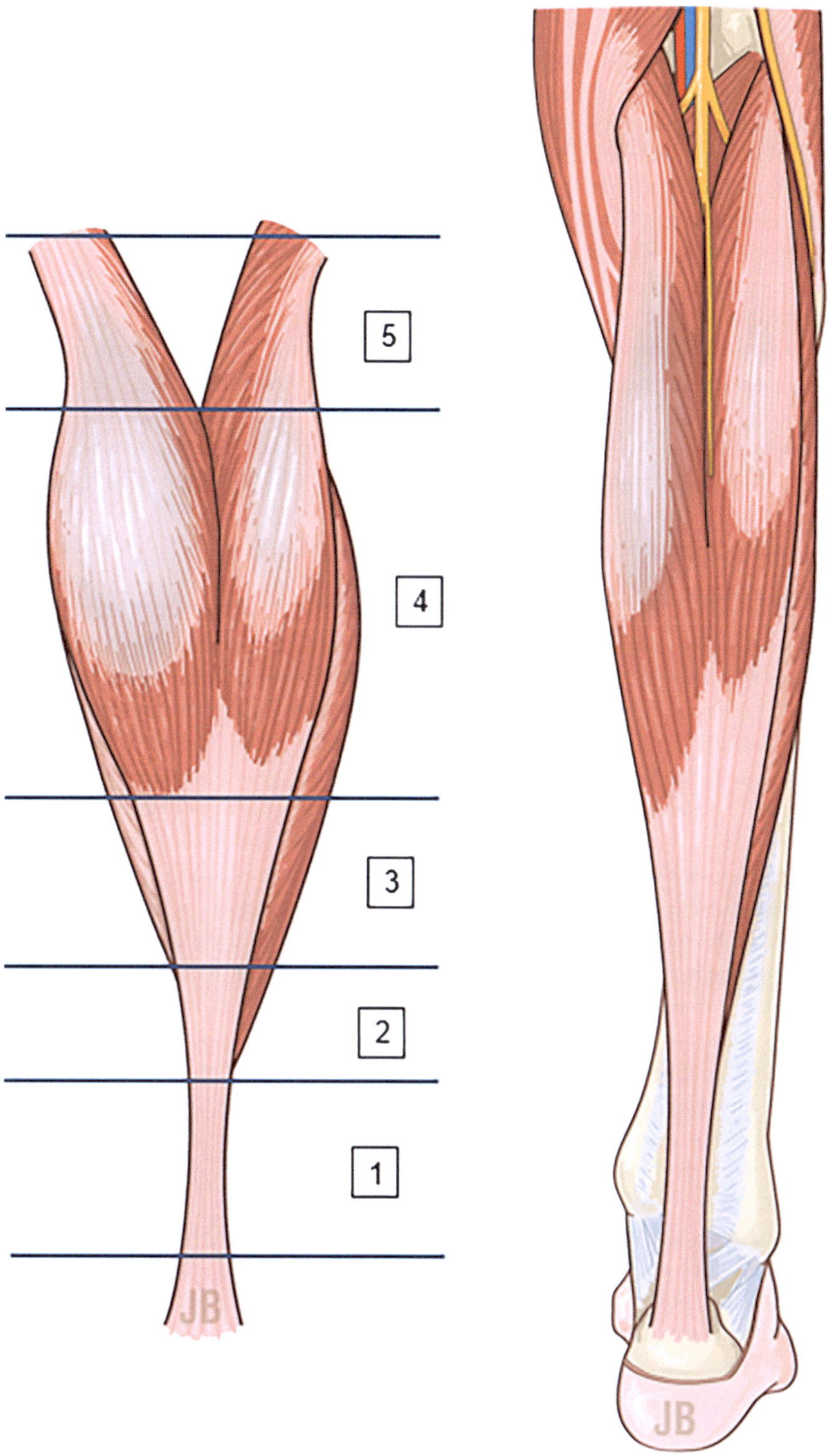

Fig. 21.1 Lengthening of gastrocnemius-soleus complex is divided in five levels

subcutaneous tissue and fascia. The procedure can be performed with a needle introduced perpendicular to the aponeurosis or with a hook blade introduced parallel through a small lateral incision [20]. Hydrodissection is necessary to create a working space between the superficial fascia and the tendinous part of the proximal gastrocnemius aponeurosis. This hydrodissection prevents lesions of the small saphenous vein. Lengthening at this level is challenging because the medial aponeurosis is curved, short, and fine; thus, a complete section requires two or three entry points [21], and the aponeurosis must be held in tension by an assistant [20, 21].

At level 4, the most significant difficulty is working in a "virtually closed space" between the anterior part of the gastrocnemius and the posterior part of the soleus muscle. Hydrodissection requires a high quantity of fluid because the space between the soleus and gastrocnemius is a real avascular space (between the knee and the middle of the leg and across the entire width of the leg). Thus, the working space at this level is not truly considered as hydrodissection. The medial portal is located under ultrasound guidance between the two belly muscles. Lengthening at this level is very safe because this space is a virtual and avascular zone. The plantaris tendon could be noted on the medial part of this space. After hydrodissection between the two aponeuroses by the medial portal, a hook knife is introduced, and the section is made from lateral to medial under ultrasound control with the probe in a transversal position [22]. Originally, this procedure was described for a section of the anterior aponeurosis of the gastrocnemius, but it could be used for a section of the posterior aponeurosis of the soleus during the same procedure by reversing the hook knife during a second pass. At this level, a section of the aponeurosis is not possible with a needle, only with an anterograde or retrograde knife.

Lengthening at levels 2 and 3 is our preference: The lengthening zone is easy to access (thin subcutaneous fatty tissue), the aponeurosis at this level is more flat and less convex than in more proximal zones, and the only structure to take care of is the sural nerve, which is easily identifiable. Depending on the width of the aponeurosis, a cutting instrument could be introduced by one or two portals on the central and medial part of the lengthening zone. A needle could be also used in perpendicular portals.

21.2.1 Our Technique

For novice sonographers, the most straightforward, reproducible, and secure lengthening technique is at level 3. At this level, the small width and flattened shape of the aponeurosis make lengthening easier. This technique ensures significant elongation potential and can be performed with a needle or any hook knife (anterograde or retrograde). It can also be realized under local anesthesia without a tourniquet.

The patient is positioned in the supine position with the foot protruding from the table.

The first step involves localizing the level of lengthening. With the ultrasound probe in a longitudinal position, we identify the distal part of the medial gastrocnemius belly muscle on the Achilles tendon. Lengthening will be located 2 or 3 cm distally to this zone (Fig. 21.2). A horizontal skin landmark is drawn at this level.

The next step is locating the sural nerve. The nerve is found in the distal third of the leg, near the ankle, lateral to the Achilles tendon, with a honeycomb pattern and close to veins. With the probe in a transverse plane, we follow the nerve proximally from the distal and lateral part of the

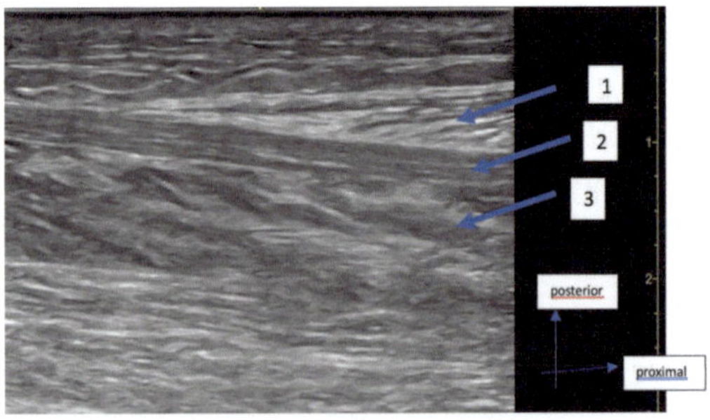

Fig. 21.2 Longitudinal section of Achilles tendon on the middle third of the leg. Lengthening is located 2 or 3 cm distally to the end of gastrocnemius muscular fibers (vertical arrow). (1) Muscular fibers of the gastrocnemius. (2) Achilles tendon. (3) Muscular fibers of the soleus

leg at the ankle to the proximal area until the level of lengthening. A vertical skin landmark is drawn at this position.

The entire foot and ankle are disinfected with povidone-iodine or chlorhexidine. A sterile cover is used for the probe (5–18 MHz), and only sterile gloves are used.

The sterile procedure begins with hydrodissection between the muscular fascia and the common aponeurosis of the gastrocnemius and soleus. This requires attention at the level of the sural nerve to prevent its lesion during lengthening. The probe is used in a transversal position, and the hydrodissection needle is introduced in an in-plane position (Fig. 21.3). Sealing the entry point with Betadine gel™ prevents air bubbles from entering and distorting the ultrasound image.

When a needle is used for the release, two or three entry points are made perpendicular to the aponeurosis. Sectioning is facilitated by tensioning the aponeurosis with dorsiflexion of the ankle by an assistant. During this release, the probe is positioned in a transversal position (in-plane from the needle), and the complete section is controlled with the probe in a longitudinal position.

When a hook knife is used, it is introduced through a medial portal inside the hydrodissection space between the aponeurosis and fascia. Cutting is controlled with the probe in a transversal position, and the complete section is monitored with the probe in a longitudinal position (section is considered complete when the hook knife can pass above and below the aponeurosis). Depending on the width of the aponeurosis and the cutting knife, one or two portals are necessary.

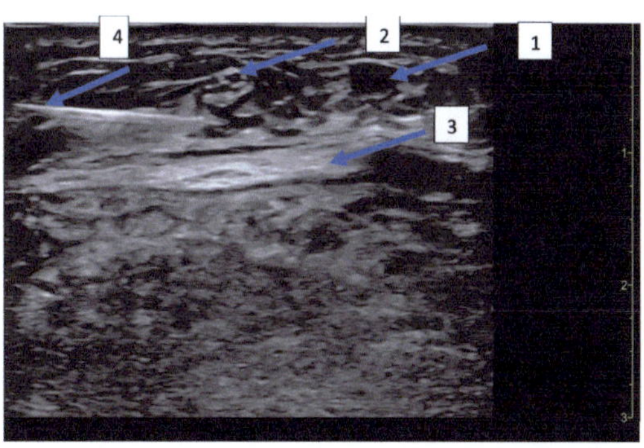

Fig. 21.3 Probe in transverse position at the level of Achilles lengthening. Hydrodissection of the sural nerve. (1) veinous (2) sural nerve (3) Achilles tendon (4) needle

Scars are closed with strips or glue.

The patient leaves the clinic walking in a boot and full weight bearing is allowed. After 2 weeks, walking is allowed with a cushioning shoe, and assisted physical or auto-administered physical therapy can begin according to specific lengthening protocols (Stanish or Alfredson). Complete resolution of pain and clinical symptoms is expected 3 months postoperatively. Return to sports is possible within the same time frame.

References

1. Dalmau-Pastor M, Fargues-Polo B, Casanova-Martínez D, Vega J, Golanó P. Anatomy of the triceps surae: a pictorial essay. Foot Ankle Clin. 2014;19(4):603–35.
2. DiGiovanni CW, Kuo R, Tejwani N, Price R, Hansen ST, Cziernecki J, et al. Isolated gastrocnemius tightness. J Bone Joint Surg Am. 2002;84(6):962–70.
3. Rosenbloom AL, Silverstein JH. Connective tissue and joint disease in diabetes mellitus. Endocrinol Metab Clin N Am. 1996;25(2):473–83.
4. Hill RS. Ankle equinus. Prevalence and linkage to common foot pathology. J Am Podiatr Med Assoc. 1995;85(6):295–300.
5. Lavery LA, Armstrong DG, Boulton AJM, Diabetex Research Group. Ankle equinus deformity and its relationship to high plantar pressure in a large population with diabetes mellitus. J Am Podiatr Med Assoc. 2002;92(9):479–82.
6. Barouk P, Barouk LS. Clinical diagnosis of gastrocnemius tightness. Foot Ankle Clin. 2014;19(4):659–67.
7. Pinney SJ, Hansen ST, Sangeorzan BJ. The effect on ankle dorsiflexion of gastrocnemius recession. Foot Ankle Int. 2002;23(1):26–9.
8. Hsu RY, VanValkenburg S, Tanriover A, DiGiovanni CW. Surgical techniques of gastrocnemius lengthening. Foot Ankle Clin. 2014;19(4):745–65.
9. Lamm BM, Paley D, Herzenberg JE. Gastrocnemius soleus recession: a simpler, more limited approach. J Am Podiatr Med Assoc. 2005;95(1):18–25.
10. Chen L, Ma X, Wang X, Huang J, Zhang C, Wang C. Comparison of four methods for percutaneous Achilles tendon lengthening: a cadaveric study. J Foot Ankle Surg Off Publ Am Coll Foot Ankle Surg. 2017;56(2):271–6.
11. Rush SM, Ford LA, Hamilton GA. Morbidity associated with high gastrocnemius recession: retrospective review of 126 cases. J Foot Ankle Surg Off Publ Am Coll Foot Ankle Surg. 2006;45(3):156–60.

12. De los Santos-Real R, Morales-Muñoz P, Payo J, Escalera-Alonso J. Gastrocnemius proximal release with minimal incision: a modified technique. Foot Ankle Int. 2012;33(9):750–4.
13. Apaydin N, Bozkurt M, Loukas M, Vefali H, Tubbs RS, Esmer AF. Relationships of the sural nerve with the calcaneal tendon: an anatomical study with surgical and clinical implications. Surg Radiol Anat SRA. 2009;31(10):775–80.
14. Sanchez PJ, Grady JF, Saxena A. Percutaneous ultrasonic tenotomy for Achilles tendinopathy is a surgical procedure with similar complications. J Foot Ankle Surg Off Publ Am Coll Foot Ankle Surg. 2017;56(5):982–4.
15. Gamba C, Serrano-Chinchilla P, Ares-Vidal J, Solano-Lopez A, Gonzalez-Lucena G, Ginés-Cespedosa A. Proximal medial gastrocnemius release versus open plantar fasciotomy for the surgical treatment in recalcitrant plantar fasciitis. Foot Ankle Int mars. 2020;41(3):267–74.
16. Chraim M, Alrabai HM, Krenn S, Bock P, Trnka HJ. Short-term results of endoscopic percutaneous longitudinal tenotomy for noninsertional Achilles tendinopathy and the presentation of a simplified operative method. Foot Ankle Spec. 2019;12(1):73–8.
17. Tennant JN, Amendola A, Phisitkul P. Endoscopic gastrocnemius release. Foot Ankle Clin. 2014;19(4):787–93.
18. Toomey EP, Seibert NR. The use of ultrasound to isolate the gastrocnemius-soleus junction prior to gastrocnemius recession. Foot Ankle Clin. 2014;19(4):739–43.
19. Agius L, Wickham A, Walker C, Knudsen J. Achilles tenotomy as an office procedure and current practising trends among New Zealand orthopaedic surgeons. N Z Med J. 2018;131(1475):44–50.
20. Villanueva M, Iborra Á, Ruiz MDM, Sanz-Ruiz P. Proximal ultrasound-guided gastrocnemius recession: a new ultra-minimally invasive surgical technique. J Foot Ankle Surg Off Publ Am Coll Foot Ankle Surg. 2019;58(5):870–6.
21. Iborra Marcos Á, Villanueva Martínez M, Fahandezh-Saddi Díaz H. Needle-based gastrocnemius lengthening: a novel ultrasound-guided noninvasive technique. J Orthop Surg. 2022;17(1):435.
22. Moroni S, Fernández-Gibello A, Nieves GC, Montes R, Zwierzina M, Vazquez T, et al. Anatomical basis of a safe mini-invasive technique for lengthening of the anterior gastrocnemius aponeurosis. Surg Radiol Anat SRA. 2021;43(1):53–61.
23. Villanueva M, Iborra Á, Rodríguez G, Sanz-Ruiz P. Ultrasound-guided gastrocnemius recession: a new ultra-minimally invasive surgical technique. BMC Musculoskelet Disord. 2016;17(1):409.

Part VII

Foot

22 Echo Surgery for Morton's Neuroma: A Minimally Invasive Approach

Benamran Lionel and Julien Beldame

22.1 Introduction

Morton's neuroma is a very painful, but frequent foot condition, which Civinini and Durlacher were the first to describe in 1845 [15], while Morton [22] gave it his name 31 years later in 1876. It mostly affects women (prevalence of 4 to 1), with a mean age of around 50 years [4, 10].

It is caused by a canal syndrome [19], where the compression of the common plantar digital nerves of medial plantar nerve causes lesions in the nerve sheath, which increases the thickness of the nerve, exacerbating the compression and the pain.

The nerve is trapped between the ground, the metatarsal heads, and under the deep transverse intermetatarsal ligament, which gives the nerve a zigzag orientation, compressing the vasa nervorum and causing ischemia. The neuroma is composed of fibrotic scar tissue surrounding the nerve due to these repeated traumas and ischemia [9].

Supplementary Information The online version contains supplementary material available at https://doi.org/10.1007/978-3-031-88679-9_22.

B. Lionel (✉)
Cabinet Archimède, Versailles, France

J. Beldame
Institut de la Cheville et du Pied Amiens, Polyclinique de Picardie, Amiens, France

Institut de la Cheville et du Pied Paris, Paris, France

22.2 Diagnosis

The diagnosis of Morton's neuroma is traditionally based on the clinical history and physical examination, as well as ultrasound, which is a very valuable tool to exclude other pain generators in the forefoot or detect unsuspected additional lesions [14].

The typical presentation includes electric shock-like pain in the third intermetatarsal space of the foot, less commonly in the second intermetatarsal space, and sometimes in both [10]. The pain radiates into the halves of the pulp of the two toes of the interspace in electric shock-like discharges. The patients often describe tingling, burning, and sometimes numbness in the area after a walk and a short relief when they massage their foot [16].

Mulder's test is a reference used in the clinical examination: if the compression of the metatarsal heads combined to compression of the painful interspace reproduces the pain, the test is considered in favor of Morton's neuroma [5, 13].

The use of ultrasound as a first-line examination can help confirm the diagnosis of Morton's neuroma and rule out other causes, such as a stress fracture of the metatarsal, lesions of the plantar plate on hyper pressure of the metatarsal heads, or Freiberg's disease while also allowing for more precise surgical indications regarding the localization of the neuroma.

O. Marès et al. (eds.), *Ultrasound-Guided Limb Surgery*,
https://doi.org/10.1007/978-3-031-88679-9_22

Using ultrasound, Morton's neuroma can be detected as a well-defined hypoechoic structure with proximal and distal continuity to the nerve and the size of the neuroma can be measured. If the ultrasound is not conclusive, an injected MRI should be offered as second-line [18].

22.3 Treatment

As with other orthopedic pathologies, conservative treatments should be prioritized. It is common to propose orthopedic insoles as a first intent, which can eventually be associated with a corticosteroid injection of the neuroma, before thinking about surgery. The orthopedic insoles include a retro capital drop to lift and spread the heads of the central metatarsals and support under the heads of the first and fifth metatarsals [1]. Ultrasound-guided injections can have good results [12] but can cause several complications, such as atrophy of the fat pad [3] of the metatarsal heads or skin depigmentation [20], or dislocations of the metatarsophalangeal joint [8]. Surgical treatment of Morton's neuroma is indicated when conservative medical treatments are not effective.

22.3.1 Surgical Management

Standard surgical techniques include neurolysis or neurectomy via plantar, dorsal, interdigital, or endoscopic approaches. Neurolysis or section of the deep transverse intermetatarsal ligament is usually the first approach, and neurectomy can be envisaged only when neurolysis fails to treat the patient [6, 21].

Neurolysis can be performed using different techniques, such as open, endoscopic, or ultrasound-guided surgery. Endoscopic decompression of the common plantar digital nerves of the medial plantar nerve proved to be much more beneficial overall than open surgery techniques. Thanks to smaller incisions, the recovery was faster with less postoperative pain and swelling and a much lower risk of infection [2, 11, 17]. Still, even with the endoscopic technique, three incisions are needed and no visualization of the nerve is possible [2].

A Spanish team described in 2020 a very promising ultrasound-guided neurolysis technique under local anesthesia, using a single 1–2 mm incision [7]. This technique uses ultrasound imaging to guide the surgeon, allowing for precise localization of the affected area, and targeted delivery of treatment. It is a minimally invasive procedure that can be done on an outpatient basis, reducing the risk of complications associated with surgery such as bleeding or infection, allowing for a quicker recovery time, with a very good level of cost efficiency compared to open surgery, obtaining favorable results in more than 98% of cases, improving dramatically over the first 3 months and continuing to improve at 6 months [7].

Because the ultrasound-guided release of the deep transverse intermetatarsal ligament is a highly precise and technically demanding procedure, it should be performed by skilled foot and ankle surgeons who have experience with ultrasound-guided procedures.

22.3.2 Personal Technique

Candidates for ultrasound-guided percutaneous release are those diagnosed with Morton's neuroma, with recalcitrant pain, unalleviated by conservative treatment.

22.3.2.1 Setup

A trowel handle is used as a countersupport under the sole of the foot to open the third interspace. The countersupport allows a perfect view of Morton's neuroma, the dorsal interosseus muscle, and the deep transverse intermetatarsal ligament (Fig. 22.1). A pad and a sterile drape are placed on it, and the foot is positioned on top, previously disinfected with chlorhexidine.

The surgeon is equipped with sterile gloves.

The ultrasound probe is introduced in a sterile cover, and sterile gel is used between the skin and the probe to avoid air interference.

The instrumentation used includes (Fig. 22.2):

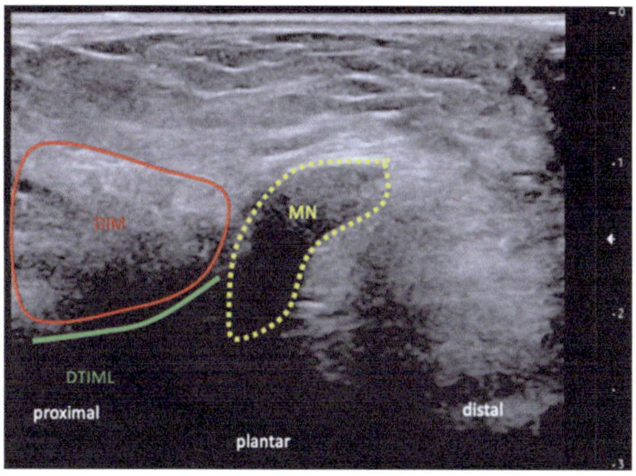

Fig. 22.1 Morton's neuroma echographic anatomy

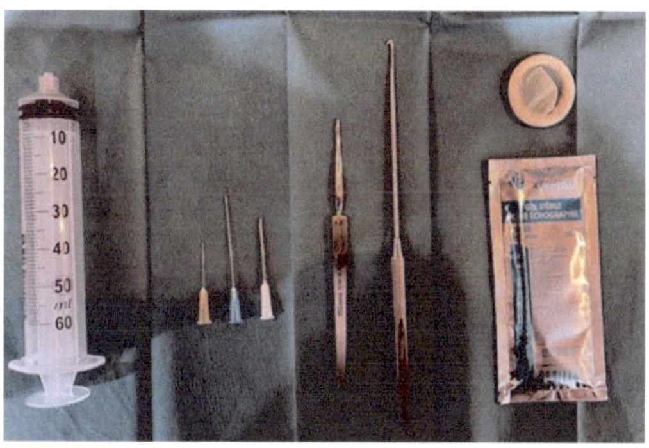

Fig. 22.2 Instrument set

- Needles: orange 25G, green 21G 50 mm, white 16G
- A 3 mm diameter hook knife
- A 1 mm blunt gouge
- A 50 ml Luer Lock syringe, sterile ultrasound gel, and a sterile probe cover

Surgery is performed under wide awake local anesthesia with 20 ml of lidocaine with epinephrine 10 mg/ml and 20 ml of 0.9% saline solution, injected under the skin between the toes in the interspace to be operated on with a 25G needle.

22.3.2.2 Surgery (Video 1)

A 21G 50-mm-long needle is introduced under ultrasound guidance to reach the distal bursa, superficial to the neuroma. The bursa is detected through progressive hydrodissection. The bursa is reached when the neuroma "descends," allowing direct access to the deep transverse intermetatarsal ligament. Local anesthesia is continued by infiltrating the deep transverse intermetatarsal ligament.

The needle hole is enlarged with a 16-gauge needle, and a 1 mm blunt gouge is introduced, passing over the neuroma and under the deep transverse intermetatarsal ligament to dissect, create a path, and identify the ligament: The blunt gouge remains well under the ligament (Fig. 22.3).

A hook is then used, following the same path, to section the ligament in a retrograde manner, ensuring that the flexor tendons are not caught in the hook – this is verified by asking the patient to move their toes (Figs. 22.4 and 22.5).

The same blunt gouge is used to verify that it passes without resistance through the deep transverse intermetatarsal ligament.

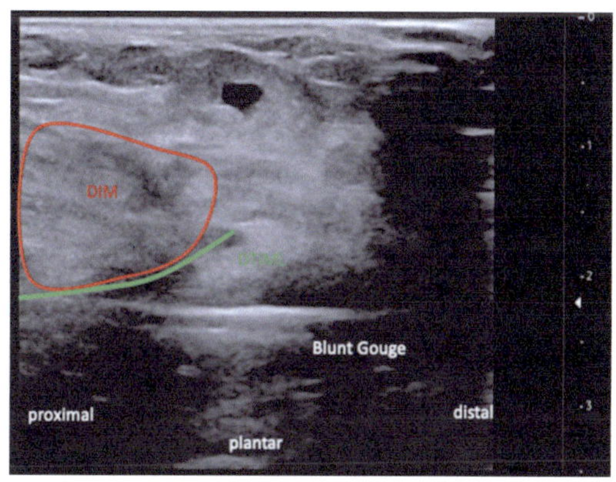

Fig. 22.3 Position of the blunt gouge

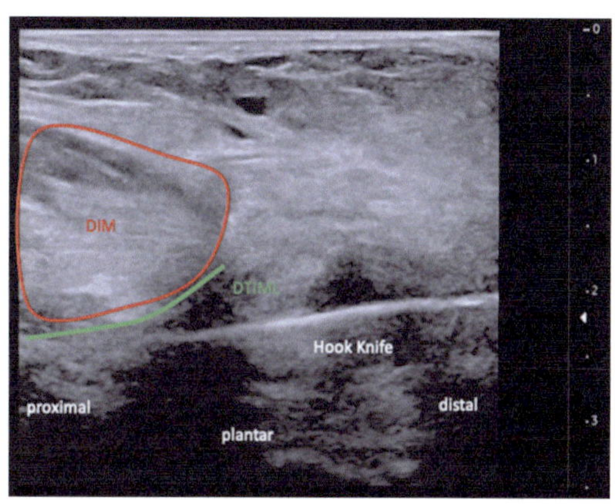

Fig. 22.4 Position of the hook knife

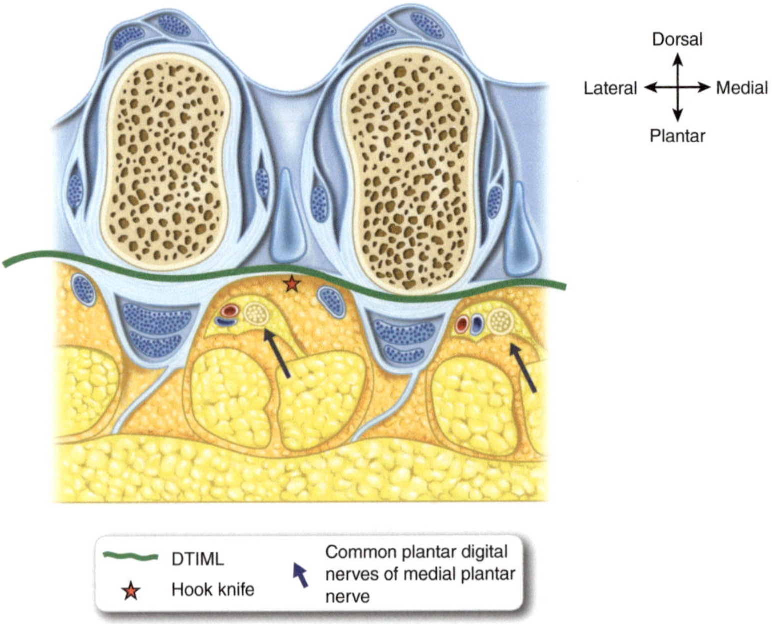

Fig. 22.5 Anatomy and the position of the hook knife

The surgical wound is not closed but covered with a small dressing.

22.3.2.3 Postoperative Care

Wound home care instructions are provided.

It is recommended to elevate the foot and apply cold for a few days. Painkillers are prescribed for postoperative pain, especially during the first days. The patients can go on with their daily routine 48 h after surgery, avoiding overuse during the first 3 weeks. A hematoma and bruising can be present for 2–5 weeks, during which Morton's neuroma is irritated and can reproduce the same symptoms.

22.4 Conclusion

In conclusion, Morton's neuroma is a painful foot condition that can be diagnosed through clinical examination and ultrasound imaging. Conservative treatments are usually the first line of treatment, but surgical intervention may be necessary. Ultrasound-guided technique has shown promising results in providing relief for patients.

Take-Home Messages

Indication

Morton's neuroma with recalcitrant pain, unalleviated by conservative treatment.

Contraindication

Patients with vascular deformity such as superficial artery or cyst.

Surgical Technique

(a) Surgery is performed under wide awake local anesthesia.
(b) The countersupport allows a perfect view of Morton's neuroma, the dorsal interosseus muscle, and the deep transverse intermetatarsal ligament.
(c) The needle hole is enlarged with a 16-gauge needle, and a 1 mm blunt gouge is introduced, passing over the neuroma and under the deep transverse intermetatarsal ligament to dissect, and create a path.
(d) A hook is then used, following the same path, to section the ligament in a retrograde manner, ensuring that the

flexor tendons are not caught in the hook.
(e) Control the release with the blunt gouge.
(f) The surgical wound is not closed but covered with a small dressing.

Postoperative care

(a) It is recommended to elevate the foot and apply cold for a few days. Painkillers are prescribed for postoperative pain.

Conclusion

Morton's neuroma is a painful foot condition that can be diagnosed through clinical examination and ultrasound imaging. Conservative treatments are usually the first line of treatment; ultrasound-guided techniques have shown promising results in providing relief for patients.

Bibliography

1. Albano D, Bonifacini C, Zannoni S, Bernareggi S, Messina C, Galia M, Sconfienza LM. Plantar forefoot pain: ultrasound findings before and after treatment with custom-made foot orthoses. Radiol Med. 2021;126:963–70. https://doi.org/10.1007/s11547-021-01354-8.
2. Barrett SL, Walsh AS. Endoscopic decompression of intermetatarsal nerve entrapment: a retrospective study. J Am Podiatr Med Assoc. 2006;96:19–23. https://doi.org/10.7547/0960019.
3. Basadonna PT, Rucco V, Gasparini D, Onorato A. Plantar fat pad atrophy after corticosteroid injection for an interdigital neuroma: a case report. Am J Phys Med Rehabil. 1999;78:283–5. https://doi.org/10.1097/00002060-199905000-00021.
4. Bradley N, Miller WA, Evans JP. Plantar neuroma: analysis of results following surgical excision in 145 patients. South Med J. 1976;69:853–4.
5. Claassen L, Bock K, Ettinger M, Waizy H, Stukenborg-Colsman C, Plaass C. Role of MRI in detection of Morton's neuroma. Foot Ankle Int. 2014;35:1002–5. https://doi.org/10.1177/1071100714540888.
6. Dellon AL. Treatment of Morton's neuroma as a nerve compression. The role for neurolysis. J Am Podiatr Med Assoc. 1992;82:399–402. https://doi.org/10.7547/87507315-82-8-399.
7. Iborra-Marcos A, Villanueva-Martinez M, Barrett SL, Sanz-Ruiz P. Ultrasound-guided decompression of the intermetatarsal nerve for Morton's neuroma: a novel closed surgical technique. J Am Podiatr Med Assoc. 2020;110:Article 8. https://doi.org/10.7547/19-033.
8. Ito E, Shima H, Togei K, Hirai Y, Tsujinaka S, Yasuda T, Neo M. Dislocations of the second and third metatarsophalangeal joints after local steroid injection in patients with refractory metatarsalgia: a case report. SAGE Open Med Case Rep. 2021;9:2050313X211046744. https://doi.org/10.1177/2050313X211046744.
9. Jain S, Mannan K. The diagnosis and management of Morton's neuroma: a literature review. Foot Ankle Spec. 2013;6:307–17. https://doi.org/10.1177/1938640013493464.
10. Kasparek M, Schneider W. Surgical treatment of Morton's neuroma: clinical results after open excision. Int Orthop. 2013;37:1857–61. https://doi.org/10.1007/s00264-013-2002-6.
11. Kubota M, Ohno R, Ishijima M, Hanyu R, Sakai K, Sugawara Y, Ochi H, Mukasa H, Kaneko K. Minimally invasive endoscopic decompression of the intermetatarsal nerve for Morton's neuroma. J Orthop. 2014;12:S101–4. https://doi.org/10.1016/j.jor.2014.01.004.
12. Lizano-Díez X, Ginés-Cespedosa A, Alentorn-Geli E, Pérez-Prieto D, González-Lucena G, Gamba C, de Zabala S, Solano-López A, Rigol-Ramón P. Corticosteroid injection for the treatment of Morton's neuroma: a prospective, double-blinded, randomized, placebo-controlled trial. Foot Ankle Int. 2017;38:944–51. https://doi.org/10.1177/1071100717709569.
13. Mahadevan D, Venkatesan M, Bhatt R, Bhatia M. Diagnostic accuracy of clinical tests for Morton's neuroma compared with ultrasonography. J Foot Ankle Surg. 2015;54:549–53. https://doi.org/10.1053/j.jfas.2014.09.021.
14. Oliver TB, Beggs I. Ultrasound in the assessment of metatarsalgia: a surgical and histological correlation. Clin Radiol. 1998;53:287–9. https://doi.org/10.1016/s0009-9260(98)80128-1.
15. Pasero G, Marson P. Filippo Civinini (1805–1844) and the discovery of plantar neuroma. Reumatismo. 2006;58:319–22. https://doi.org/10.4081/reumatismo.2006.319.
16. Pastides P, El-Sallakh S, Charalambides C. Morton's neuroma: a clinical versus radiological diagnosis. Foot Ankle Surg. 2012;18:22–4. https://doi.org/10.1016/j.fas.2011.01.007.
17. Shapiro SL. Endoscopic decompression of the intermetatarsal nerve for Morton's neuroma. Foot Ankle Clin. 2004;9:297–304. https://doi.org/10.1016/j.fcl.2003.12.004.

18. Unger HR, Mattoso PQ, Drusen MJ, Neumann CH. Gadopentetate-enhanced magnetic resonance imaging with fat saturation in the evaluation of Morton's neuroma. J Foot Surg. 1992;31:244–6.
19. Vachon P, Lemay M, Bouchard HL. Pathologic study of Morton's neuroma. Can J Surg. 1991;34:356–8.
20. Vasile G, Hosseinipour M, Hoffman C, Gropper C. Linear depigmentation after an intralesional corticosteroid injection. J Clin Aesthet Dermatol. 2020;13:49–51.
21. Villas C, Florez B, Alfonso M. Neurectomy versus neurolysis for Morton's neuroma. Foot Ankle Int. 2008;29:578–80. https://doi.org/10.3113/FAI.2008.0578.
22. The Classic. A peculiar and painful affection of the fourth metatarso-phalangeal articulation, vol. 142. Thomas G. Morton, M.D. Clin Orthop Relat Res; 1979. p. 4–9.

23 Plantar Fasciitis

R. Sacco, L. Mebarki, and J. Beldame

23.1 Introduction

Plantar fasciitis, also known as plantar fasciopathy, is a condition that causes heel pain due to microtears in the plantar fascia, a band of connective tissue that runs from the heel to the toes. These microtears result from repetitive stress and lead to chronic degenerative changes at the proximal attachment of the plantar fascia to the calcaneus.

23.2 Anatomy and Physiology

The plantar fascia (PF) consists of three parts: medial, central, and lateral (Picture 23.1). The PF originates from the medial tubercle of the calcaneus proximally and extends distally to cover the plantar surface of the foot. It then splits into five slips that insert into the capsules of the metatarsophalangeal joints (MTPJs) and the proximal phalanges of the toes.

- The central part is the thickest and most prominent part of the PF. It covers the plantar surface of the flexor digitorum brevis muscle and inserts into the MTPJs of the toes.
- The lateral part covers the plantar surface of the abductor digiti minimi muscle and inserts into the MTPJ of the fifth toe.
- The medial part is the thinnest and less distinct part of the PF. It covers the plantar surface of the abductor hallucis muscle and inserts into the MTPJ of the first toe [1].

Histologically, the PF is mainly composed of type I collagen fibers that are oriented in a proximal-distal direction. Immunohistochemical staining reveals numerous nerve endings and proprioceptive corpuscles, especially on the inner surface [1], suggesting that the PF may play a role in proprioception, control, and stability of foot movements.

The PF has two main functions: supporting the foot arch and facilitating the windlass mechanism. When the foot is weight-bearing, the PF prevents the foot arch from collapsing by acting as a tension band. During walking, when the MTPJs dorsiflex, the PF tightens and increases the height of the foot arch, creating a rigid lever for propulsion [2].

The relationship between the PF and the Achilles tendon (AT) is controversial. Although the PF and the AT share a common embryological origin, anatomical studies have not consistently

R. Sacco
Centre Hospitalier de Rouen Universitaire de Rouen, Rouen, France

L. Mebarki
Centre Médical International de Monaco, Monaco, Monaco

J. Beldame (✉)
Institut de la Cheville et du Pied Amiens, Polyclinique de Picardie, Amiens, France

Institut de la Cheville et du Pied Paris, Paris, France

O. Marès et al. (eds.), *Ultrasound-Guided Limb Surgery*,
https://doi.org/10.1007/978-3-031-88679-9_23

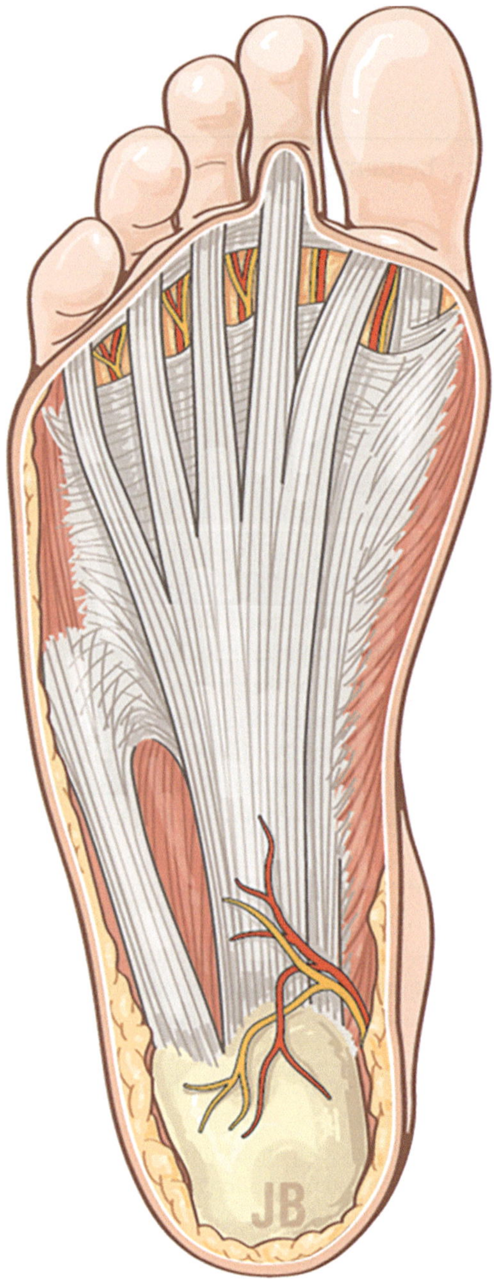

Picture 23.1 Dissection view of the plantar aponeurosis: after resection of the cutaneous tissue, visualization of the plantar aponeurosis after section. (Courtesy of Dr. Lisa Mébarki, Monaco)

found direct fibrous connections between them [3]. However, these two structures are anatomically and physiologically linked by soft tissue connections, such as the calcaneal periosteum [4].

23.3 Overview

PF is the most common cause of heel pain in adults, affecting 10% of the US population [5]. The pathogenesis of PF involves degeneration and inflammation caused by micro-injuries at the bone-tendon junction of the calcaneus [6]. The main symptom of PF is heel pain, which is worsened by walking, exercising on hard surfaces, or standing for prolonged periods [7, 8].

Plantar fasciitis (PF) is more prevalent among women, middle-aged patients, long-distance runners, soldiers, obese patients, patients with either pes cavus (high-arched), pes planus (flat) foot deformity, or limited ankle dorsiflexion [7, 8]. Conservative treatment is the first-line therapy for PF, with 90% of patients undergoing rest, nonsteroidal anti-inflammatory drugs (NSAIDs), stretching, plantar orthosis, corticosteroid injection, extracorporeal shockwave therapy, and ultrasound therapy [9]. The use of analgesics is the most common treatment, accounting for 47% of all treatments, while exercise counseling and physical therapy account for 26% and 19%, respectively [9]. If heel pain persists after 12 months of conservative treatment, surgery may be indicated.

23.4 Imaging

The diagnosis of plantar fasciitis, which is primarily based on clinical examination in the presence of plantar heel pain, is confirmed by medical imaging techniques. The most common differential diagnoses are irritation of Baxter's nerve (inferior calcaneal nerve), tarsal tunnel syndrome, and insertional tendinopathy of the Achilles tendon. Radiographs are the first diagnostic imaging modality and allow the evaluation of conditions such as a tumor, fracture, and calcaneal spurs, although magnetic resonance imaging (MRI) and ultrasonography (US) have advantages in directly evaluating the plantar fascia [10]. PF is associated with the presence of calcaneal spurs on X-ray, with spur length and base width being associated with pain level; on the other hand, spurs have been also detected in many painless feet [11]. MRI or ultrasound can show a thickened plantar fascia, with an increment of the thickness of the plantar aponeurosis of 1.62 mm for blinded studies and up to 2.20 mm for unblinded studies [12]. A meta-analysis revealed that patients with PF were 634 times more likely to have a plantar fascia thickness greater than 4 mm when compared with healthy controls. The presence of hypoechogenicity on ultrasound and hyperintensity of signal on MRI are significantly associated with PF. At more advanced stages, the presence of plantar fascia tears can be found [12]. Sonoelastography studies suggest a loss of elasticity associated with PF, sometimes in isolation without other plantar fascia changes [13]. Sonoelastography is not yet performed in current clinical practice, but this technique has a promising role in the early diagnosis of PF.

23.5 Surgical Treatment (Tables 23.1 and 23.2)

Plantar fasciotomy is considered as the surgical treatment of reference [14]. However, several studies have found better outcomes and higher patient satisfaction rates with the proximal gastrocnemius recession compared to the open plantar fasciotomy [15, 16]. Radiofrequency tenotomy [17] showed similar results when compared with various different surgical interventions, including open fasciotomy [18], endoscopic fasciotomy [19], and proximal gastrocnemius release [20]. Dry needling has the advantage of being a minimally invasive technique, but it has demonstrated significant clinical improvement only compared to corticosteroid injection [21] and extracorporeal shockwave therapy [22].

Significant better results was seen in endoscopic procedure than open technique during the first three month [23, 24]. According to Catal et al. [25], a superficial approach with an endoscopic portal on the plantar side of the PF is associated with a significant clinical improvement at 3 weeks, with faster operative time and fewer complications. It is recommended to opt for a partial fasciotomy of the medial half or two-thirds of the plantar fascia during plantar fasciotomy, to avoid changes in the morphologic and functional characteristics of the foot [26, 27]. However, some studies did not report significant Djian-Annonier's angle modification after total fasciotomy [28].

Table 23.1 Percutaneous procedures without ultrasound control

Bermejo et al. [30]	Longitudinal tenotomy	Technical note	
Catal et al. [29]	Percutaneous fasciotomy with needle	Anatomical study	On the middle part of the aponeurosis
Colberg et al. [32]	Percutaneous 40 skin punctures with 18-gauge needle	40 patients Local tibial block	At the level of the calcaneal insertion
Benton-Weil et al. [33]	Percutaneously by beaver-blade	51 patients Local anesthesia	At the level of the calcaneal insertion

Table 23.2 Percutaneous techniques with ultrasound control

Iborra et al. [31] (2021)	Partial fasciotomy with local tibial block 16-gauge needle	107 patients	Heel pain improved in 92.5% No complication
Vohra and Japour [34] (2009)	Intervenous and local anesthesia With tourniquet Retrograde knife	46 feet/41 patients	No complication
Malahias et al. [35] (2022)	Local anesthesia V-lance knife	15 patients	Two patients with refractory neuropathic pain over the lateral border of the foot

Overall, percutaneous procedures may differ according to the orientation, location, and extent of the plantar fasciotomy. Percutaneous techniques are generally associated with a transverse fasciotomy [29] and have the advantage of being performed under local anesthesia without a tourniquet (Wide-Awake Local Anesthesia No Tourniquet, "WALANT"). In contrast, Bermejo et al. [30] have suggested that a longitudinal fasciotomy, similar to the treatment for Achilles tendinitis, could "allow the patient to quickly resume their activities."

Ultrasound-guided plantar fasciotomy is a newer approach that avoids damage to the muscles, lateral plantar nerve, and Baxter's nerve. Iborra et al. [31] conducted a relevant study that involved 107 patients undergoing tibial nerve anesthesia. The procedure, which lasted 10–15 min, involved a fasciotomy of 50% of the width of the PF on the medial side, and did not require any suture. No nerve complications, vascular injuries, or wound-related problems were recorded during a follow-up period up to 24 months. The authors emphasized the reduced cost of their procedure and the patients' ability to return to work quickly. Other studies have reported good or excellent results using different types of surgical instruments.

23.6 Our Surgical Technique

Our technique is similar to the procedure described by Iborra et al. [31].

- The patient is placed in a supine position with the affected limb in external rotation, and the foot placed at the end of the examination table (Picture 23.2).
- The procedure begins with local anesthesia (xylocaine 1%) of the tibial nerve at the posteromedial part of the medial malleolus under ultrasound control. For the local anesthesia, we routinely use specific needles with foam edges to prevent nerve lesions.
- A sterile surgical field is prepared at the time of the patients' installation for the anesthesia. The whole foot and ankle are disinfected with povidone-iodine or chlorhexidine. A sterile cover is used for the probe (5–18 MHz), and only sterile gloves are used.

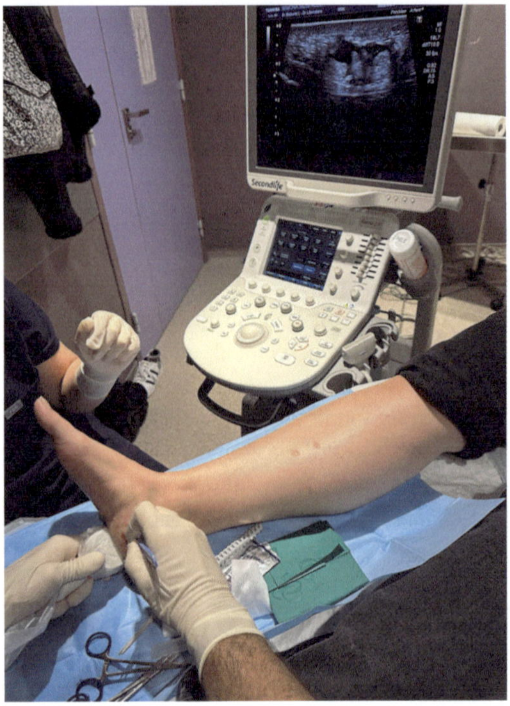

Picture 23.2 Longitudinal view ultrasound at the plantar level. The chamber of dissection is realized under direct control with ultrasound. (Courtesy of Dr. Lisa Mébarki, Monaco)

- A syringe with 20 cc of ropivacaine 2% with a 22-gauge needle is used to make a chamber of dissection on the plantar, superficial side of the aponeurosis (hydrodissection). The probe is positioned longitudinally, and the needle is introduced on the medial side of the heel. A chamber of dissection between the plantar fat pad and the aponeurosis is very useful to achieve an optimal visualization of the plantar aspect of the PF (Picture 23.3). During hydrodissection, the probe is placed on a transverse position to follow the hydrodissection from the medial to the lateral side of the aponeurosis.
- With the probe in a longitudinal orientation, the hydrodissection is then performed on the deep side of the aponeurosis. This is very important to prevent neurologic or vascular lesions during the section of the plantar fascia.
- When hydrodissection is accomplished on both sides of the aponeurosis (superficial

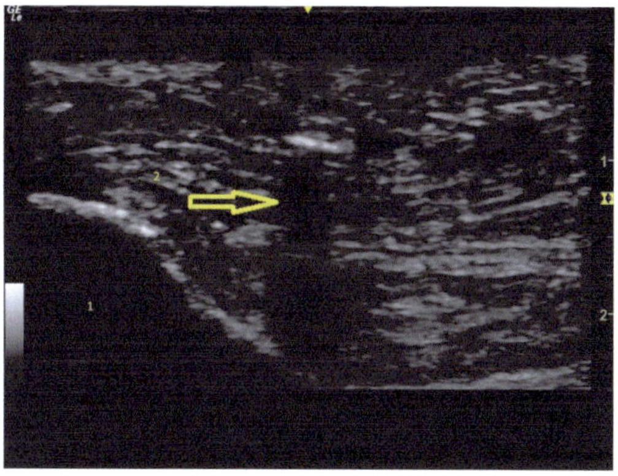

Picture 23.3 An ultrasound image showing a cross-sectional view of tissue with varying shades of gray. A prominent yellow arrow points to a specific area, possibly indicating a region of interest or abnormality. The image includes numerical labels "1" and "2" near the arrow. A grayscale bar is visible on the left, and measurement markers are on the right side. The texture suggests a medical examination, possibly of soft tissue

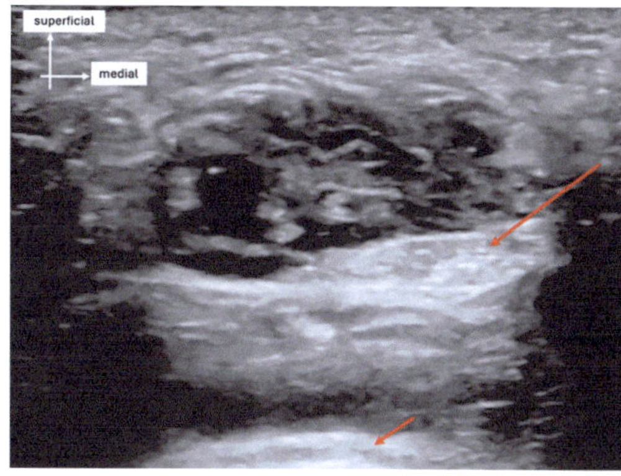

Picture 23.4 Transverse view after hydrodissection. The long arrow corresponds to the medial part of the aponeurosis, the short arrow corresponds to the calcaneal cortex

and deep), the medial half of the aponeurosis is sectioned. The section is performed 2 or 3 cm distally to the calcaneal insertion of the plantar fascia. Sealing the entry point with Betadine gel™ prevents air bubbles from entering and distorting the ultrasound image.

– A mini skin incision of 2 or 3 mm on the medial side of the heel is followed by retrograde introduction of a knife under the aponeurosis. A small incision is important to maintain a certain amount of pressure in the chamber of hydrodissection and keep a proper visualization during the section of the aponeurosis.
– The knife is introduced under the aponeurosis, between the fat pad and the aponeurosis, with the probe kept in a transverse orientation (Picture 23.4). The knife is introduced until it reaches the medial half of the aponeurosis, and then the section is made by retrograde traction. The section is controlled on longitudinal and transverse positions of the probe, while the knife can move from the plantar to the deep side of the aponeurosis. The number of times that the knife needs to be passed to section the PF is influenced by the thickness of the aponeurosis. The wound is closed with glue or is sutured if larger than 4 mm. It is possible to inject 1 cc of dexamethasone or platelet-rich plasma (PRP) to reduce local inflammation and pain.

The patient leaves the clinic walking full weight bearing in a boot. After 2 weeks, walking is allowed with a cushioning shoe. Some patients may benefit from physical therapy. Complete resolution of pain and clinical symptoms is expected 3–6 months postoperatively. Return to sport is possible within the same time frame.

In our experience we did not encounter any nervous or vascular complications. Residual pain after percutaneous echographic surgery may require additional infiltrations, such as PRP, when inflammation persists. Plantar orthosis can be used between the third and the sixth month.

Take-Home Message

Indication

Patient with surgery indications for the plantar fasciitis

After the failure of the medical treatment

The patient must have a normal rear foot

Contraindication

Patients with rear foot deformity

(continued)

Surgical Technique

WALANT anesthesia 30/50 cc; at the lower part of the medial part of the distal tibia

Transverse view of the insertion of the plantar fascia at the calcaneum level

Find the best entry point with a 22-Gauge needle on a transverse view. The probe should be 1 cm up the junction between the plantar skin on the medial side of the foot. And 2 cm distal from the insertion at the calcaneum level.

The anesthesia should create at this moment a place to work with the knife

Open the skin with a knife on 2 or 3 mm

Hydrodissection is made on both side of the aponevrosis

Then, the knife is inserted; it should engage the whole plantar fascia

The section is done on an in-plane view to control the full or partial release of the fascia; it depends on the author

Postoperative care

Pressure dressing for 48 h

Protective splint 10 days and progressive recovery.

Conclusion

Ultrasound release of the plantar fascia is feasible with this mini-invasive technique. The first results are interesting. The risk of deformity of the rear foot should be noticed for patient with flat feet and for full section of their PF.

References

1. Stecco C, Corradin M, Macchi V, Morra A, Porzionato A, Biz C, et al. Plantar fascia anatomy and its relationship with Achilles tendon and paratenon. J Anat. 2013;223(6):665–76.
2. Chen D, Wei LB, Aubeeluck A, Feng YY, Gang HY, Qian ZJ, et al. Anatomy and biomechanical properties of the plantar aponeurosis: a cadaveric study. PLoS One. 2014;9(1):e84347.
3. Kim PJ, Richey JM, Wissman LR, Steinberg JS. The variability of the Achilles tendon insertion: a cadaveric examination. J Foot Ankle Surg Off Publ Am Coll Foot Ankle Surg. 2010;49(5):417–20.
4. Singh A, Zwirner J, Templer F, Kieser D, Klima S, Hammer N. On the morphological relations of the Achilles tendon and plantar fascia via the calcaneus: a cadaveric study. Sci Rep. 2021;11(1):5986.
5. Ahn J, Yeo J, Lee SH, Lee YJ, Park Y, Goo B, et al. Healthcare usage and cost for plantar fasciitis: a retrospective observational analysis of the 2010-2018 health insurance review and assessment service national patient sample data. BMC Health Serv Res. 2023;23(1):546.
6. Goff JD, Crawford R. Diagnosis and treatment of plantar fasciitis. Am Fam Physician. 2011;84(6):676–82.
7. Cutts S, Obi N, Pasapula C, Chan W. Plantar fasciitis. Ann R Coll Surg Engl. 2012;94(8):539–42.
8. Thompson JV, Saini SS, Reb CW, Daniel JN. Diagnosis and management of plantar fasciitis. J Am Osteopath Assoc. 2014;114(12):900–6.
9. Riddle DL, Schappert SM. Volume of ambulatory care visits and patterns of care for patients diagnosed with plantar fasciitis: a national study of medical doctors. Foot Ankle Int. 2004;25(5):303–10.
10. Lareau CR, Sawyer GA, Wang JH, DiGiovanni CW. Plantar and medial heel pain: diagnosis and management. J Am Acad Orthop Surg. 2014;22(6):372–80.
11. Okçu M, Tuncay F, Koçak FA, Erden Y, Ayhan MY, Kaya SS. Do the presence, size, and shape of plantar calcaneal spurs have any significance in terms of pain and treatment outcomes in patients with plantar fasciitis? Turk J Med Sci. 2023;53(1):413–9.
12. Drake C, Whittaker GA, Kaminski MR, Chen J, Keenan AM, Rathleff MS, et al. Medical imaging for plantar heel pain: a systematic review and meta-analysis. J Foot Ankle Res. 2022;15(1):4.
13. Lee SY, Park HJ, Kwag HJ, Hong HP, Park HW, Lee YR, et al. Ultrasound elastography in the early diagnosis of plantar fasciitis. Clin Imaging. 2014;38(5):715–8.
14. Nayar SK, Alcock H, Vemulapalli K. Surgical treatment options for plantar fasciitis and their effectiveness: a systematic review and network meta-analysis. Arch Orthop Trauma Surg. 2023;143(8):4641–51.
15. Gamba C, Serrano-Chinchilla P, Ares-Vidal J, Solano-Lopez A, Gonzalez-Lucena G, Ginés-Cespedosa A. Proximal medial gastrocnemius release versus open plantar fasciotomy for the surgical treatment in recalcitrant plantar fasciitis. Foot Ankle Int. 2020;41(3):267–74.
16. Monteagudo M, Maceira E, Garcia-Virto V, Canosa R. Chronic plantar fasciitis: plantar fasciotomy versus gastrocnemius recession. Int Orthop. 2013;37(9):1845–50.
17. Chou ACC, Ng SYC, Su DHC, Singh IR, Koo K. Radiofrequency microtenotomy is as effective as plantar fasciotomy in the treatment of recalcitrant plantar fasciitis. Foot Ankle Surg Off J Eur Soc Foot Ankle Surg. 2016;22(4):270–3.

18. Yuan Y, Qian Y, Lu H, Kou Y, Xu Y, Xu H. Comparison of the therapeutic outcomes between open plantar fascia release and percutaneous radiofrequency ablation in the treatment of intractable plantar fasciitis. J Orthop Surg. 2020;15(1):55.
19. Wang W, Rikhraj IS, Chou ACC, Chong HC, Koo KOT. Endoscopic plantar fasciotomy vs open radiofrequency microtenotomy for recalcitrant plantar fasciitis. Foot Ankle Int. 2018;39(1):11–7.
20. Huang DM, Chou AC, Yeo NE, Singh IR. Radiofrequency microtenotomy with concurrent gastrocnemius recession improves postoperative vitality scores in the treatment of recalcitrant plantar fasciitis. Ann Acad Med Singap. 2018;47(12):509–15.
21. Uygur E, Aktaş B, Eceviz E, Yilmazoğlu EG, Poyanli O. Preliminary report on the role of dry needling versus corticosteroid injection, an effective treatment method for plantar fasciitis: a randomized controlled trial. J Foot Ankle Surg Off Publ Am Coll Foot Ankle Surg. 2019;58(2):301–5.
22. Rahbar M, Eslamian F, Toopchizadeh V, Jahanjoo F, Kargar A, Dolatkhah N. A Comparison of the Efficacy of Dry-Needling and Extracorporeal Shockwave Therapy for Plantar Fasciitis: A Randomized Clinical Trial. Iran Red Crescent Med J [Internet]. 29 sept 2018 [cité 29 Oct 2023]; (In Press). Disponible sur: https://archive.ircmj.com/article/20/9/ircmj-20-9-68908.pdf
23. Chou ACC, Ng SYC, Koo KOT. Endoscopic plantar fasciotomy improves early postoperative results: a retrospective comparison of outcomes after endoscopic versus open plantar fasciotomy. J Foot Ankle Surg Off Publ Am Coll Foot Ankle Surg. 2016;55(1):9–15.
24. Feng SM, Song RL, Wang AG, Sun QQ, Zhang SC. Endoscopic partial plantar fasciotomy via 2 medial portals vs mini-open procedure for refractory plantar fasciitis. Foot Ankle Int. 2021;42(4):458–63.
25. Çatal B, Keskinbora M, Uysal MA, Şahin M, Gulabi D, Demiralp B. Endoscopic plantar fasciotomy; deep fascial versus superficial fascial approach: a prospective randomized study. J Foot Ankle Surg. 2017;56(5):1001–8.
26. Johannsen F, Konradsen L, Hansen P, Brinch S, Nybing JU, Krogsgaard MR. The effect of endoscopic partial plantar fasciotomy on morphologic and functional properties of the foot. Foot Ankle Int. 2023;44(5):415–23.
27. Murphy GA, Pneumaticos SG, Kamaric E, Noble PC, Trevino SG, Baxter DE. Biomechanical consequences of sequential plantar fascia release. Foot Ankle Int. 1998;19(3):149–52.
28. Maes R, Safar A, Ghistelinck B, Labadens A, Hernigou J. Percutaneous plantar fasciotomy: radiological evolution of medial longitudinal arch and clinical results after one year. Int Orthop. 2022;46(4):861–6.
29. Çatal B, Keskinbora M, Keskinöz EN, Tümentemur G, Azboy İ, Demiralp B. Percutaneous plantar fascia release with needle: anatomic evaluation with cadaveric specimens. J Foot Ankle Surg Off Publ Am Coll Foot Ankle Surg. 2019;58(5):842–6.
30. Bermejo M, Lucar-López G, Ballester-Alomar M, Córdoba-Fernández A, Martínez-Souto C, Villamizar M, et al. Ultrasound-guided longitudinal tenotomy for plantar fasciitis. Technical note and systematic review. Acta Ortop Mex. 2022;36(4):252–6.
31. Iborra A, Villanueva M, Sanz-Ruiz P, Martin A, Noriega C. A novel closed technique for ultrasound-guided plantar fascia release with a needle: review of 107 cases with a minimum follow-up of 24 months. J Orthop Surg. 2021;16(1):153.
32. Colberg RE, Kenneth-Nwosa KO, Jurado Vélez JA, Slowik JS, Fleisig GS. Clinical and imaging outcomes of plantar fasciotomy using microdebrider coblation wand. Foot Ankle Orthop. 2022;7(2):24730114221091797.
33. Benton-Weil W, Borrelli AH, Weil LS, Weil LS. Percutaneous plantar fasciotomy: a minimally invasive procedure for recalcitrant plantar fasciitis. J Foot Ankle Surg Off Publ Am Coll Foot Ankle Surg. 1998;37(4):269–72.
34. Vohra PK, Japour CJ. Ultrasound-guided plantar fascia release technique: a retrospective study of 46 feet. J Am Podiatr Med Assoc. 2009;99(3):183–90.
35. Malahias MA, Roumeliotis L, Tyrpenou E, Kazas ST, Sourlas I, Kaseta MK. Ultrasound-guided partial plantar fascia release with the use of a fine cutting device for the treatment of persistent plantar fasciitis: a case series. J Am Podiatr Med Assoc. 2022;112(2):20–244.

Part VIII

Green Surgery

24 Quality of Carpal Tunnel Surgery: The Impact of Ultrasound Surgery and Office Practice

Olivier Marès, Lara Moscato, and Pascal Kouyoumdjian

24.1 Introduction

Wide-awake local anesthesia with no tourniquet (WALANT) has become an increasingly popular alternative to locoregional anesthesia (LRA) [1] for carpal tunnel release. Ultrasound-guided surgery and local anesthesia have enabled this type of procedure to be performed outside the operating room, in an outpatient department [2] with many advantages that have already been reported in the literature [3].

24.2 Study

We compared 3 care pathways using 3 groups of 30 patients each:

- Ultrasound-guided WALANT surgery in office surgery with simplified draping (EcWO)
- Ultrasound-guided surgery under WALANT in an outpatient unit without anesthetic monitoring (EcWA)
- Endoscopic surgery under LRA in the main OR, with monitoring and tourniquet (EnAA)

O. Marès (✉) · P. Kouyoumdjian
Department of Traumatology and Orthopedics Surgery, University Hospital Nîmes, Nîmes, France

L. Moscato
CHU de Montpellier, Montpellier, France

The same surgeon performed all procedures. All procedures performed under WALANT used the US-guided anterograde release technique with a Kemis® knife (NewClip® Technics, France) [4]. Endoscopic releases were performed under LRA using the Agee technique [5].

LRA anesthesia was performed by an anesthesiologist with ultrasound guidance, monitoring, and intravenous sedation. WALANT anesthesia was performed by the surgeon 15–20 min before incision, using an equivalent solution of sodium bicarbonate and lidocaine +1% epinephrine, and did not require monitoring.

The "office surgery" procedure took place in an outpatient department assisted by a trained nurse and used a reduced sterile drape.

Surgery in the operating room was carried out using a conventional "extremity drape." A tourniquet was applied to the arm for LRA procedures.

Satisfaction was rated from 0 (complete disappointment) to 10 (complete satisfaction), for each criterion:

- Overall satisfaction with care
- Concerning the conditions in which the operation was carried out
- Concerning the quality of anesthesia
- Concerning the conditions under which the anesthesia was performed

O. Marès et al. (eds.), *Ultrasound-Guided Limb Surgery*,
https://doi.org/10.1007/978-3-031-88679-9_24

We found by comparing the three pathways that there is a significative improvement in overall satisfaction when the procedure is carried out in office surgery compared with management in the operating theater ($p = <0.0001$) (Table 24.1).

On the anesthesia aspect, we found that WALANT provided superior satisfaction compared with LRA regarding the quality of anesthesia ($p = 0.0014$).

Thereafter, we carried out 1-to-1 analyses of overall satisfaction and satisfaction with the quality of anesthesia, the results of which are shown in Table 24.2. We found no significant difference in the quality of anesthesia between the office surgery and WALANT ambulatory groups. This result was expected since the quality of WALANT anesthesia is not influenced by the place where it's performed.

On the other hand, we highlighted a significant difference between the LRA group and the two WALANT groups with increased satisfaction in the WALANT groups, which shows that the type of anesthesia plays a major role in patient satisfaction.

All patients experienced a disappearance of paresthesias regardless of the surgical technique used, with no significant difference ($p = 0.8401$). This result shows the same security of the ultrasound technique compared to the Agee technique.

Our study seems to show an improvement in overall satisfaction with the use of WALANT and US-guided surgery compared with locoregional anesthesia and endoscopic management. Patients treated with WALANT seemed to be more satisfied with the office surgery than with the conventional care in the operating room.

Carpal tunnel release was initially performed under general anesthesia in the operating room [5]. Practices have evolved with the evolution of techniques and are in line with patients' expectations and preferences in terms of management and care pathways [6, 7]. WALANT [8] has proven its efficacy in terms of analgesia [9], has excellent patient tolerance [10, 11], and offers numerous advantages for both the surgeon [12–14] and the healthcare system in general [15].

This type of anesthesia has made it possible to relocate this kind of surgical procedure outside the operating room without any increase in complications [16–18], without any alteration in the postoperative clinical outcome [19], with a reduction in costs [20] and a clear reduction in the time required for patient care [21].

The benefits of minimally invasive anesthetic management and office surgery are well established in the literature. Administered in restricted doses [22, 23], local anesthesia does not require intravenous drip administration or monitoring, nor does it require pre-anesthetic consultation or the services of an anesthesiologist. Unlike LRA, there was no need for post-anesthetic monitoring in a care unit, which helped to reduce the time spent by the patient in the care facility. No preoperative fasting was required, nor was there any need to adapt or temporarily stop the patient's treatments. Performing a surgical procedure in an office surgery seems to strengthen the patient-surgeon relationship and thus appears to contribute to increased patient compliance [24, 25].

Allowing patients to talk to their surgeon throughout the procedure helps to significantly reduce anxiety, as does the absence of massive,

Table 24.1 Comparison of satisfaction data from the three groups using a numerical analog scale

Satisfaction: mean score (from 0 to 10)	EcWO	EcWA	EnAA	*p*-value
Overall satisfaction	9.87	9.37	8.60	< 0.00001
Pathway satisfaction	9.87	9.63	9.63	0.2716
Anesthesia performance satisfaction	9.37	9.53	8.87	0.0918
Anesthesia quality satisfaction	9.93	9.93	9.40	0.0014

Table 24.2 Group-by-group comparison of overall satisfaction and satisfaction with anesthesia quality

Comparison	Overall satisfaction Mean difference	*p* value	Anesthesia quality satisfaction Mean difference	*p* value
EcWO vs. EcWA	+ 0.50	0.0292	0	0.599
EcWO vs. EnAA	+ 1.27	0.0245	+ 0.53	0.0050
EcWA vs. EnAA	+ 0.77	0.0245	+ 0.53	0.0112

occluding drapes or wearing hospital gowns. All these points help to explain the increase in patient satisfaction with the minimally invasive pathway highlighted by our study.

Although this study shows promising results, we must acknowledge a few limitations.

First, it's a retrospective study, and we will be keen to implement a prospective, randomized protocol in future studies. In addition, the presence of a recall bias, due to the heterogeneity of the delay between contact and postoperative data collection, must be acknowledged. We also acknowledge the presence of scale bias. Indeed, despite the use of an objective measurement tool such as the numerical analog scale, the perception, interpretation, and transposition of satisfaction via such a tool by the patient remain subjective and differ from one person to another.

Despite these limitations, we have nonetheless highlighted promising avenues for future work, notably concerning the importance of draping and the type of anesthesia in the patient's perception of their care [26].

24.3 Conclusion

The use of ultrasound guidance surgery under WALANT for managing carpal tunnel syndrome has shown to increase satisfaction rates and improve the perception of anesthesia quality when compared to endoscopic management under LRA. These benefits were even more pronounced when the surgery was performed in an office setting as opposed to a traditional operating room. Furthermore, there were no significant differences in clinical outcomes or increased risk of complications between the two techniques. This less invasive, more resource-efficient, and simpler approach has numerous advantages for carpal tunnel surgery, benefiting both the healthcare system and the patients' objective experience.

Ultrasound-guided WALANT surgery for carpal tunnel syndrome yields higher satisfaction and improved anesthesia perception than endoscopic LRA management, particularly in-office settings.

References

1. Lalonde D. Conceptual origins, current practice, and views of wide awake hand surgery. J Hand Surg Eur. 2017;42:886–95.
2. Lecoq B, Hanouz N, Morello R, Jean-Jacques PY, Dutheil J, Hulet C, et al. Ultrasound-assisted surgical release of carpal tunnel syndrome: results of a pilot open-label uncontrolled trial conducted outside the operating theatre. Joint Bone Spine. 2015;82:442–5.
3. Duquette S, Nosrati N, Cohen A, Munshi I, Tholpady S. Decreased wait times after institution of office-based hand surgery in a veterans administration setting. JAMA Surg. 2015;150:182–3.
4. Harris A, Meerwijk E, Kamal R, Sears E, Hawn M, Eisenberg D. Variation in surgeons requests for general anesthesia when scheduling carpal tunnel release. Hand NY; 2019. [1558944719828006]
5. Elmaraghy MW, Hurst LN. Single-portal endoscopic carpal tunnel release: Agee carpal tunnel release system. Ann Plast Surg. 1996;36:286–91.
6. Peters B, Giuffre J. Canadian trends in carpal tunnel surgery. J Hand Surg. 2018;43(1035):e1–8.
7. Munns J, Awan H. Trends in carpal tunnel surgery: an online survey of members of the American society for surgery of the hand. J Hand Surg. 2015;40:767–71.e2.
8. Lied L, Borchgrevink G, Finsen V. Wide awake hand surgery. J Hand Surg Asian Pac. 2017;22:292–6.
9. Tang JB, Gong KT, Xing SG, Yi L, Xu JH. Wide-awake hand surgery in two centers in China: experience in Nantong and Tianjin with 12,000 patients. Hand Clin. 2019;35:7–12.
10. Gunasagaran J, Sean E, Shivdas S, Amir S, Ahmad T. Perceived comfort during minor hand surgeries

with wide awake local anesthesia no tourniquet (WALANT) versus local anesthesia (LA)/tourniquet. J Orthop Surg. 2017;25:2309499017739499.
11. Teo I, Lam W, Muthayya P, Steele K, Alexander S, Miller G. Patients' perspective of wide-awake hand surgery—100 consecutive cases. J Hand Surg Eur. 2013;38:992–9.
12. Pires Neto P, Moreira L, Casas P. Is it safe to use local anesthesia with adrenaline in hand surgery? WALANT technique Rev Bras Orto. 2017;52:383–9.
13. Hagert E, Lalonde D. Time to bury the adrenaline-myth!–safe use of adrenaline anesthesia in hand surgery and orthopedics. Lakartidningen. 2015;112:C4MC.
14. Mckee D, Lalonde E, Thoma D, Dickson H. Achieving the optimal epinephrine effect in wide awake hand surgery using local anesthesia without a tourniquet. Hand. 2015;10:613–5.
15. Alter TH, Warrender WJ, Liss FE, Ilyas AM. A cost analysis of carpal tunnel release surgery performed wide awake versus under sedation. Plast Reconstr Surg. 2018;142:1532–8.
16. Tang J. Wide-awake primary flexor tendon repair, tenolysis, and tendon transfer. Clin Orthop Surg. 2015;7:275–81.
17. Lalonde D, Martin A. Wide-awake flexor tendon repair and early tendon mobilization in zones 1 and 2. Hand Clin. 2013;29:207–13.
18. Jagodzinski N, Ibish S, Furniss D. Surgical site infection after hand surgery outside the operating theatre: a systematic review. J Hand Surg Eur. 2017;42:289–94.
19. Leblanc MR, Lalonde DH, Thoma A, Bell M, Wells N, Allen M, et al. Is main operating room sterility really necessary in carpal tunnel surgery? A multicenter prospective study of minor procedure room field sterility surgery. Hand. 2011;6:60–3.
20. Kazmers N, Presson A, Xu Y, Howenstein A, Tyser A. Cost implications of varying the surgical technique, surgical setting, and anesthesia type for carpal tunnel release surgery. J Hand Surg. 2018;43:971–7.e1.
21. Van Demark R, Becker H, Anderson M, Smith V. Wide-awake anesthesia in the in-office procedure room: lessons learned. Hand N Y. 2018;13:481–5.
22. Rosenberg PH, Veering BT, Urmey WF. Maximum recommended doses of local anesthetics: a multifactorial concept. Reg Anesth Pain Med. 2004;29:564–75.
23. Yelnik A, Hentzen C, Cuvillon P, Allart E, Bonan I, Boyer F, et al. French clinical guidelines for peripheral motor nerve blocks in a PRM setting. Ann Phys Rehabil Med. 2019;62:252–64.
24. Menendez M, Chen N, Mudgal C, Jupiter J, Ring D. Physician empathy as a driver of hand surgery patient satisfaction. J Hand Surg. 2015;40:1860–5.e2.
25. Lalonde D, Martin A. Tumescent local anesthesia for hand surgery: improved results, cost-effectiveness, and wide-awake patient satisfaction. Arch Plast Surg. 2014;41:312–6.
26. Barone MM, Cogliandro A, Coppola M, Persichetti P. Role of patient-reported outcomes measures in plastic surgery. Plast Reconstr Surg. 2017;140:362e–3e.

MIX
Papier aus verantwortungsvollen Quellen
Paper from responsible sources
FSC® C105338

If you have any concerns about our products,
you can contact us on
ProductSafety@springernature.com

In case Publisher is established outside the EU,
the EU authorized representative is:
Springer Nature Customer Service Center GmbH
Europaplatz 3, 69115 Heidelberg, Germany

Printed by Libri Plureos GmbH
in Hamburg, Germany